LIVING WITH A HYPERACTIVE CHILD

An indisposable guide for helping parents and teachers to cope with hyperactivity

It's natural, it's my health

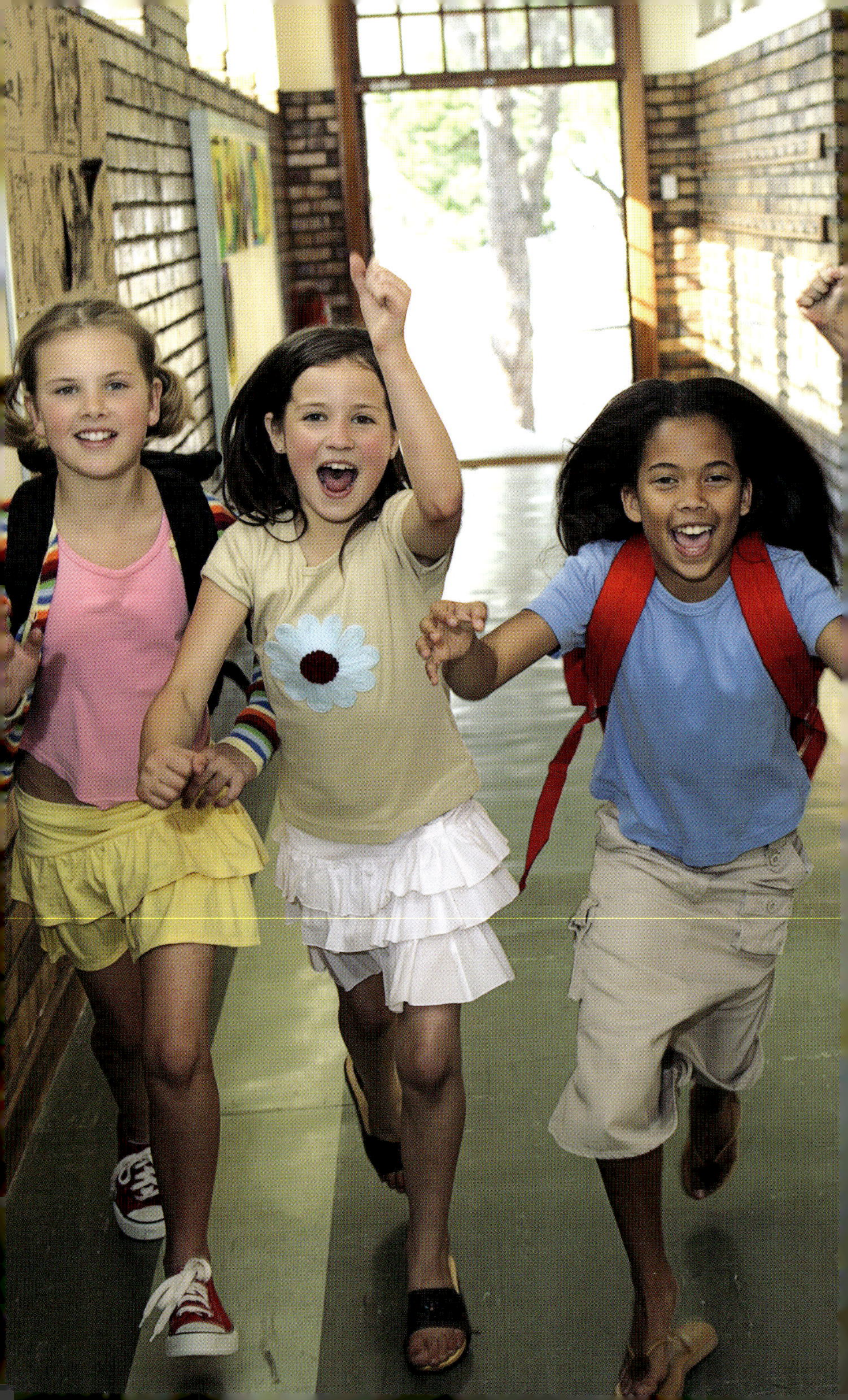

LIVING WITH A HYPERACTIVE CHILD

An indispensable guide for helping parents and teachers to cope with hyperactivity

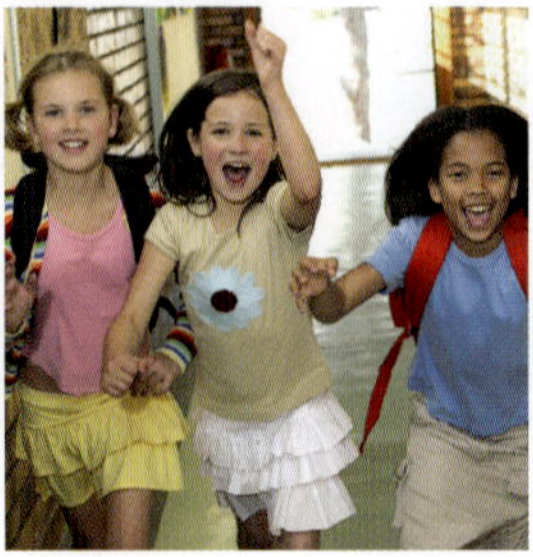

Dr Céline Causse

Editions Alpen

Alpen Éditions
9, avenue Albert II
98000 Monaco

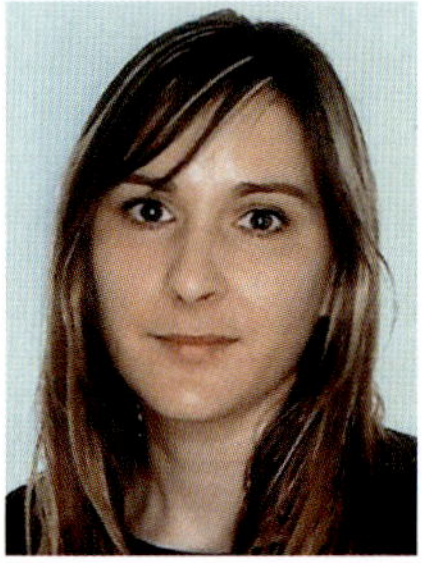

Céline Causse is a doctor and medical journalist. She is the author of a dissertation on hyperactivity, and wanted to contribute clear information on a subject which is often unclear.

NOTE:
The information contained in this book cannot replace an authoritative opinion. Before embarking on any self-medication, consult a doctor or a qualified pharmacist.

9, avenue Albert II
98000 Monaco
Tel: +377 97 77 62 10
Fax: +377 97 77 62 11
web: www.alpen.mc
e-mail: didierlaurent@alpen.mc

Printed in Canada
ISBN: 978-2-916784-20-5
UPC: 0 10043 01139 0

Introduction

Hyperactivity in children is of increasing interest as witnessed by the growing number of articles, books or television programs which have recently been dedicated to the subject. The increased frequency of the disorder, new advances in neuropsychological research, new brain imaging methods and new treatments on the market may be some of the possible explanations for this interest.

Nevertheless, hyperactivity in children continues to be a controversial subject, particularly in the United States. Historically there have been two differing schools of thought: one, which is Anglo-Saxon, defends the idea that it is a neurologically related disorder and the other, more European opinion, believes that hyperactivity is a symptom of underlying psychological problems. At present, most authors recognize hyperactivity as a separate disorder and research on its causes are pursued at different levels. The most studied issues include genetic, neurobiological and developmental factors.

Hyperactivity in children, now known as ADHD (attention deficit hyperactivity disorder) is defined by specialists by grouping three main symptoms: hyperactivity, attention deficit and impulsiveness. These are frequently associated with other disorders called "accompanying disorders": mood disorders, conduct disorders, tics, anxiety, etc. But each child is unique and hyperactivity may manifest itself differently from one child to the next. It is often difficult to establish a diagnosis since all hyperactivity is not a symptom of ADHD. However a precise diagnosis is essential for starting adequate treatment. This is often associated with behavior, counseling and medication measures. One of the medications available in the United States is methylphenidate (Ritalin® or Concerta®). The use of stimulants for treating children with ADHD is the subject of a controversy that shows no signs of ending. Much criticized and much praised, this drug is far from being universally accepted and some doctors still refuse to prescribe it.

How is hyperactivity diagnosed? Does a test exist for a sure diagnosis? Does hyperactivity disappear when the child becomes an adolescent? What is going on in the brain of a hyperactive child? What role does diet play? Is Ritalin® dangerous? These are some of the questions this book tries to answer.

Foreword *by Barbara Levenstein*

One of the many joys of parenthood is watching their baby grow and develop into a happy, well-adjusted and well-behaved child, adolescent and teen. A child who performs well in school, socializes and interacts positively with peers, family members and others is what most parents wish for their child. Many parents though, do not have the pleasure of experiencing this joy because their child suffers from Attention Deficit Hyperactivity Disorder (ADHD), a learning disability or a mood disorder. According to the National Institute of Mental Health, ADHD is one of the most common mental disorders that develop in children. It is a condition that becomes apparent in young children, but can last into adulthood, and is characterized by inattentive, hyperactive and impulsive behavior which the child can not control.

ADHD is a difficult condition to diagnose and requires a thorough examination by a qualified healthcare professional. Parents need to seek guidance from specialists to help them determine what is age-appropriate behavior and what is not, and how to manage, treat and cope with a child that suffers from ADHD. If ADHD is not addressed, the consequences for the child and family can be devastating. It is not uncommon for parents to feel guilty and blame themselves for their child's problem, and parent-child and sibling relationships are often strained.

According to CDC (Centers for Disease Control), in 2003 an estimated 4.4 million children between the ages of 4-17 were diagnosed with ADHD by a healthcare professional, and as of 2003, 2.5 million were receiving medication treatment for the disorder.

Is ADHD being over-diagnosed? What causes ADHD and how do you know if your child truly suffers from it? Where should a parent turn for guidance and what type of professional support is available? What are the treatment options? What role do diet and nutritional supplements play?

We, at Arkopharma/Health From The Sun, a company that provides nutritional support for a healthy body and mind from infancy to old age, are proud to be associated with Living With A Hyperactive Child, a book that will answer these questions and many more you may have about ADHD. This exceptional book provides an objective and in-depth look at ADHD and available options for treating, managing and coping with this disorder. If you have a child with ADHD or one you suspect may have ADHD, Living With A Hyperactive Child will help you better understand and manage this condition, and enable you to make the best choices for you, your child and your entire family.

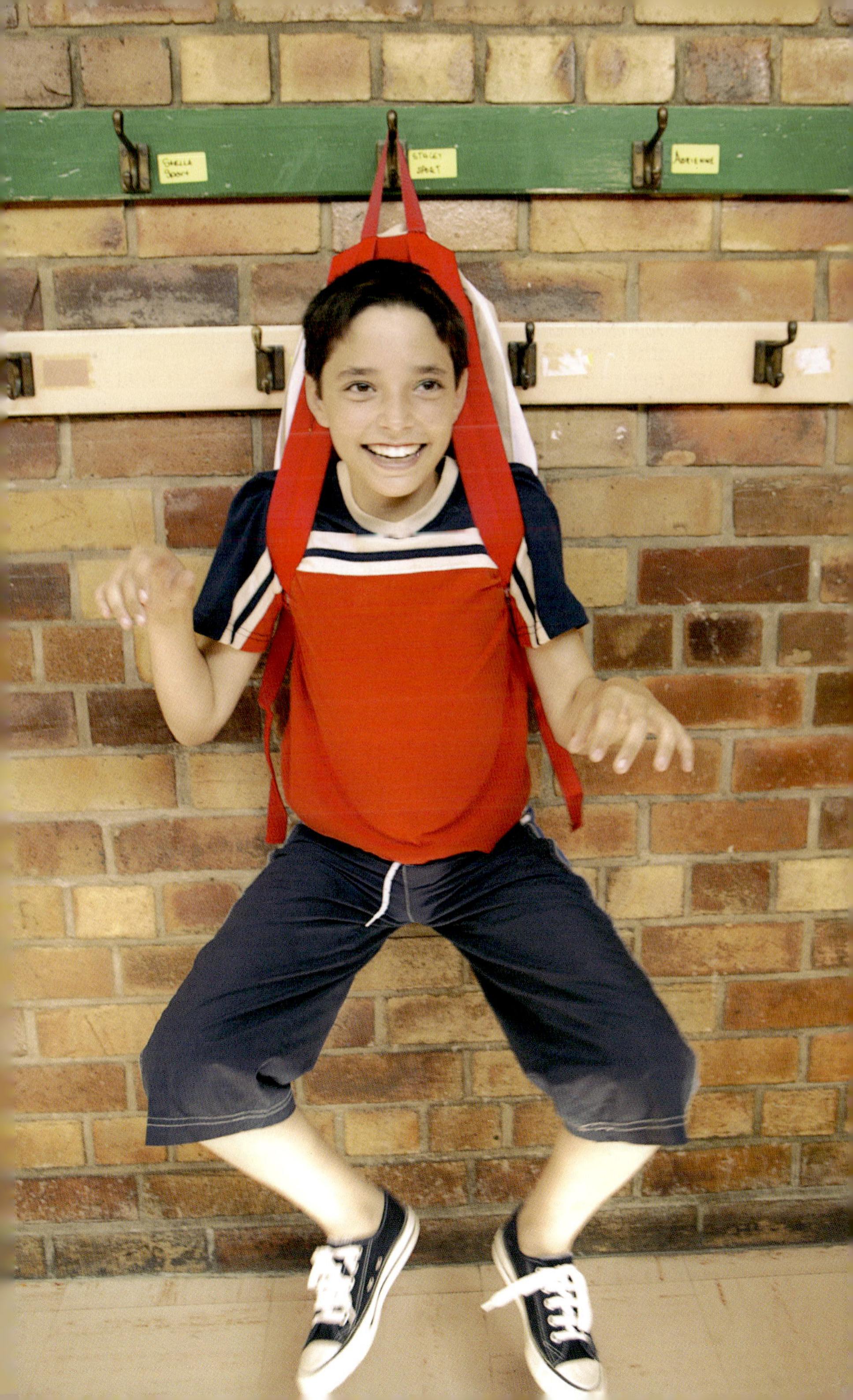

TABLE OF CONTENTS

HYPERACTIVITY, A RECOGNIZED DISORDER

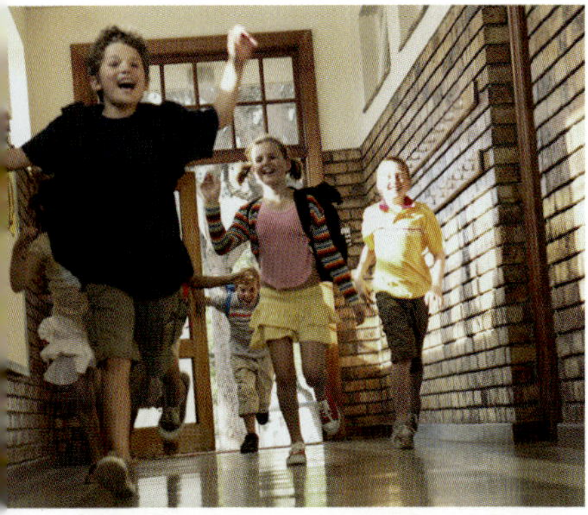

When is hyperactivity abnormal?

Talking about ADHD in children is always a subject for debate. Actually, hyperactivity is not always the symptom of a disorder, all the more so when a child is young.

Hyperactivity: a symptom or disorder?

In medicine, a symptom is a clinical sign where the causes may be multiple, unlike a disease where all the symptoms are linked to the same cause. For example, a temperature is a symptom which may be due to numerous illnesses. The flu is an illness which can be broken down into specific symptoms used to make a diagnosis. Hyperactivity was long considered by doctors as a symptom, for example of depression. We now know that hyperactivity associated with an attention deficit is a full-fledged disorder most likely of a neurological origin.

Hyperactivity is not necessarily abnormal

Moving, jumping, running, walking, playing and making noise are normal behaviors for children. They are also signs of good physical and mental health. Up until the age of three or four, children are often unruly and this is completely normal. So, making a diagnosis of hyperactivity in the pathological sense of the word is not easy at that age. In addition, confirming that a child is hyperactive when he or she is not may prove to be just as harmful as missing a real case of hyperactivity. Thus the diagnosis is often made afterward, when the hyperactivity continues past age seven *(see page 26)*.

When hyperactivity becomes pathological

Hyperactivity can be described as pathological in children when they **move constantly**, are always restless, and cannot keep themselves from moving even when doing things they like. They cannot sit quietly to draw or do homework. They endanger themselves without being aware of it. This hyperactivity is **disorderly**: they flit illogically from one activity to another. These particular actions make it possible to differentiate between pathological and commonplace hyperactivity, the latter of which is normal, despite the excessiveness. Hyperactivity becomes a real disorder, when it **interferes with the quality of life of children** and when it only causes suffering and no advantages. Most of the time, this hyperactivity is accompanied by concentration and attention disorders. Thus this set of symptoms is referred to as ADHD *(attention deficit hyperactivity disorder)*.

Hyperactivity / impulsiveness criteria

Children must have at least six out of the nine criteria below for a period of more than six months and to a degree significant enough to harm their development.

• **Hyperactivity criteria**

- often movement of hands and feet, or fidgeting when sitting
- getting up often in class or in other situations when they are supposed to be sitting
- often running or climbing everywhere in situations where it is inappropriate (afterwards in adolescents or adults, this symptom may be limited to a subjective feeling of motor impatience)
- often have a hard time staying calm while playing or during recreation activities
- are often “on the go” or act like they are “wound up like a top”
- often talk too much

• **Impulsiveness criteria**

- often blurt out the answer to a question that has not been finished being asked
- often have a hard time waiting their turn
- often interrupt others or impose their presence (for example: interrupt during conversations or games)

Source: DSM IV (Diagnostic and Statistical Manual of Mental Disorders)

Are all restless children hyperactive?

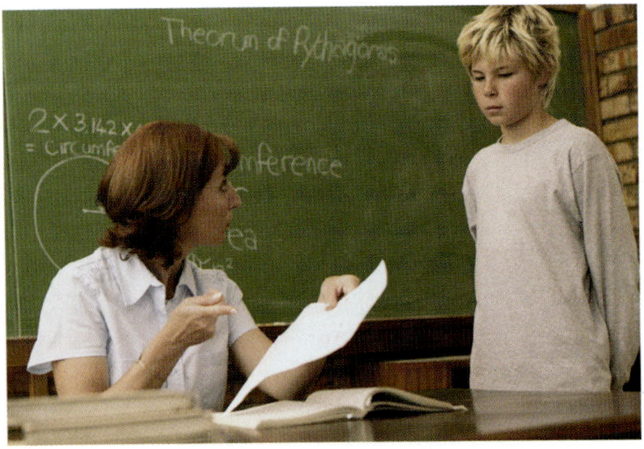

Hyperactivity, restlessness, agitation, instability, ADHD *(Attention Deficit Hyperactivity disorder)* are terms often used to describe children with exaggerated motor activity. Nevertheless they are not synonyms and only ADHD is recognized as a real disorder.

A question of vocabulary

In the United States we use hyperactivity and ADHD interchangeably, but this is a misuse of the terms that leads to confusion. Calling children hyperactive implies that they have ADHD and this is not always true. Hyperactivity is too vague a term for describing these children. It refers more to a type of behavior while the expression ADHD means a disorder with a probable neurological origin *(see page 14)*. For the sake of convenience, based on American studies on ADHD and to prevent repeating the terms, "hyperactivity" and "hyperactive children" will be used in this book to describe ADHD and the people afflicted with it. The expression "ADHD child" will also be used for the same reason.

Restlessness or ADHD?

It is not always easy to distinguish between ADHD and "simple" restlessness. The boundary between normal and pathological is sometimes fuzzy and depends on the tolerance of the environment: household, school, etc. The first questions to ask yourself, if your child is restless, are: does your child have attention problems, is he or she often absent-minded, doesn't concentrate at school or have learning disabilities due to this inattentiveness? If you answered yes to all these questions and this has been going on for several months, then it is likely your child has ADHD. Actually, in ADHD hyperactivity is generally associated with attention deficit. In some cases, there is no hyperactivity but only an attention deficit. In all cases a doctor's opinion is needed to make a diagnosis.

ADHD, an exact diagnosis

The word "hyperactivity" conceals a particular disorder, ADHD, and its diagnosis requires precise criteria. Thank goodness, every restless child does not have ADHD. Diagnosing ADHD in a child is the realm of specialists. First it is necessary to eliminate all other possible causes of hyperactivity *(see the box)*. ADHD is not the only cause for hyperactivity in children. Some hyperactivity is simply behavior related. There are children who are hyperactive, bad mannered, often aggressive or impulsive, and quick-tempered because they lack boundaries due to insufficient parental authority. Psychomotor instability may also be the result of psychological disorders. This accounts for a child's suffering or that of one of the parents, which needs to be searched for. Most often it involves a depression or conflict between the parents. In this case the instability is generally more marked at home and less at school.

Causes of hyperactivity in children unrelated to ADHD

Possible causes of psychomotor agitation in children:

- Physical causes:

- Certain neurological disorders: aftereffects of brain injuries, brain tumors, head injuries, fragile X syndrome, West's syndrome and certain forms of epilepsy.
- Hyperthyroidism.
- Reactions to some medicines: theophylline (asthma drug), barbiturates, corticoids and certain epilepsy treatments.
- Undetected vision or hearing disorders.
- Mental retardation.

- Psychological causes:

- Psychotic disorders and autistic disorders
- Early bipolar disorder (see the box on pages 22 – 23)
- Disruptive family environment and lack of child rearing
- Children who have been victims of abuse (child abuse or sexual abuse)

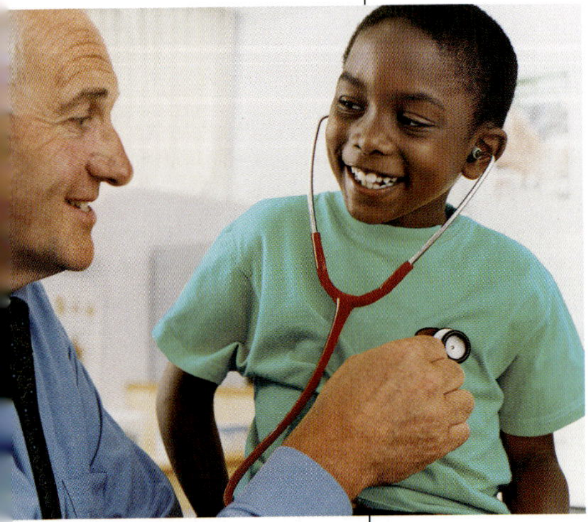

What is ADHD?

Attention deficit hyperactivity disorder, or ADHD is a neurobehavioral disorder which includes three major types of symptoms present in varying degrees: attention deficit, hyperactivity and impulsiveness.

The different ADHD subtypes

- **Combined type**: when signs of hyperactivity/impulsiveness and signs of inattention are present all at the same time and with the same intensity.
- **Predominantly inattentive type**: when attention disorders and learning disabilities are predominant.
- **Predominantly hyperactive-impulsive type**: when hyperactivity, impulsiveness and often behavior problems are predominant.

Diagnosing ADHD

To find out if your child has ADHD you need to consult a specialist, child psychiatrist or child neurologist. These assessments are usually done in three steps:

- The doctor takes a **detailed history** of the child's life since birth (has he or she had any particular illnesses, operations, how was he or she as an infant), school records (it is a good idea to bring the child's school file) and also on the entire family (are others hyperactive in the family? How was the father or uncle at the same age? Are there any particular diseases in the family?).
- Next the child is given a **complete physical**, primarily to look for minor neurological signs that are sometimes present in ADHD.
- The doctor then prescribes any **additional tests** which help to reach a diagnosis: psychological assessments, speech examination, psychomotor examination, etc.

A diagnosis will not be made until all these tests have been performed in order to be as certain as possible of the diagnosis.

International diagnostic criteria

These have been defined by international experts in DSM IV, the Diagnostic and Statistical Manual of Mental Disorders. To make a diagnosis the following are required:

- The presence of a certain number of hyperactivity or impulsivity symptoms *(see the box on pages 10-11)* as well as an inattention disorder *(see the box on pages 16-17)* present for at least six months.
- These symptoms must involve a significant change in the child's life at school, at home and in social settings.
- They must not be due to another physical or psychological disease.

Using this type of assessment may prevent certain diagnostic errors, but there is no certain sign or biological test that can be used for a 100% accurate diagnosis.

All children are different

The symptoms vary greatly from one child to the next, and in the same child over time, based on the place and circumstances. For example, one child may have significant hyperactivity, while another mainly an attention deficit. And one may be permanently hyperactive while another only occasionally. Moreover, in some children there are also associated disorders called "accompanying disorders": anxiety, tics, mood disorders, etc.

ADHD in figures

- 3-5% of children are afflicted with hyperactivity.
- 5 boys have ADHD for every girl.
- Hyperactivity is one of the leading reasons for contacting a child psychiatrist.
- Hyperactivity usually appears between age three and four.
- It is generally diagnosed around age six-seven when children start elementary school.
- 30-50% of hyperactive children will have learning disabilities.
- 20-30% of untreated hyperactive children will get into trouble with the law during adolescence.

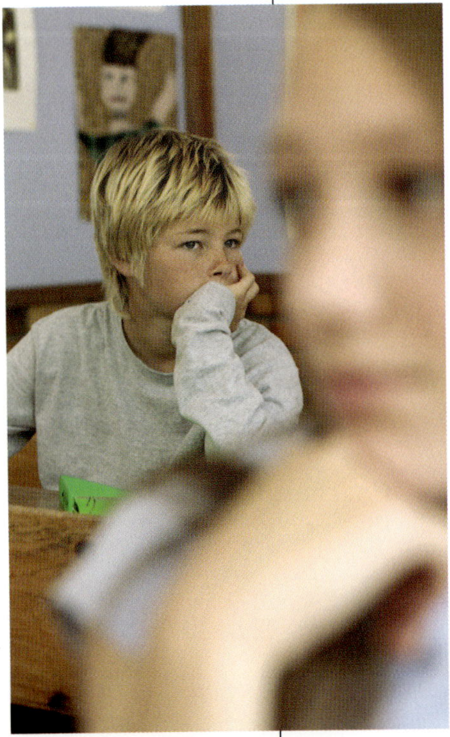

Attention deficit, an ADHD symptom

For most of us paying attention is a given. However, there are children who have a difficult, even impossible, time concentrating. This is referred to as attention deficit.

Paying attention is not always easy!

Paying attention implies being able to "forget" everything going on around you and concentrate on what you are doing. For example, in a classroom it means concentrating on your paper and ignoring your classmates, what's going on in the hall, the teacher writing on the board, and even the thoughts which pop into your head.

This ability to concentrate depends on numerous factors. Everyone knows that the level of concentration varies naturally throughout the day: it is better in the morning than in the afternoon. The pace in younger classes is adopted to fit this.

How is inattention in ADHD children manifested?

- The children are considered dreamers, have their heads in the clouds, primarily at school, but also elsewhere.
- They are often distracted by what is around them
- They seem not to be listening when called or spoken to directly
- They often forget their belongings.

All inattentive children are not hyperactive

An attention deficit is not necessarily a symptom of ADHD. There are children who daydream more than others without this being a sign of a disorder. We have all experienced the feeling of being someplace else at some time in our life, and not being able to concentrate and we are not necessarily hyperactive. Certain psychological disorders may also lead to an attention disorder in children. For example depression (which may be difficult to detect in children) or even anxiety.

Attention deficit in ADHD

Often less visible than hyperactivity, attention disorders are just as debilitating for children with ADHD. These children have a hard time following instructions, are easily distracted and cannot concentrate on a book for more than ten minutes. In addition, they won't sit still, and get out of their chairs without stopping, even when threatened with punishment. This behavior is stronger than the children: despite their willingness, they are unable to act differently. Precise criteria have been established to diagnose attention deficit *(see the box)*.

Official inattention criteria

The child must have six of the nine criteria (inappropriate for his or her development level), some of these symptoms must have appeared before the age of seven:

- Often does not give close attention to details or makes careless mistakes in schoolwork, work, or other activities.
- Often has trouble keeping attention on tasks or play activities.
- Often does not seem to listen when spoken to directly.
- Often does not follow instructions and fails to finish activities, not due to oppositional behavior or failure to understand instructions.
- Often has trouble organizing activities.
- Often avoids things that take a lot of mental effort for a long period of time (such as schoolwork or chores).
- Often loses things for school or toys.
- Is often easily distracted by exterior stimuli.
- Is often distracted or forgetful in daily activities.

Learning disabilities

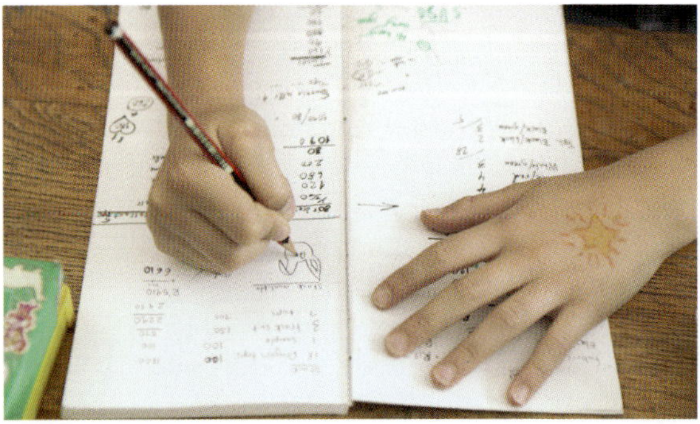

Despite a normal or even above-average intelligence, around 50% of hyperactive children have or will have learning disabilities during their school years compared with only 5% of school age children.

The problems of hyperactive children usually start in first grade, when learning to read. Discovering disorders in children as early as possible is essential in order to effectively help them and limit their falling behind which becomes worse as the months and years pass.

Discovering reading disabilities

ADHD children have a particular way of reading that is easy to detect by paying attention. They read very slowly and with great effort. It is hard for them to remember what they have read and they often don't understand the meaning. Actually, all of their attention is focused on deciphering the text and they cannot concentrate on reading and the meaning of the text at the same time. During dictation they often forget letters or words due to their attention deficit. Their writing is also particular and irregular; it appears careless, with crossing-out and scribbling. Even more importantly, it is not due to a

The different learning disabilities

Based on the disabilities discovered in the child, they are referred to as:

- **Dyslexia:** a reading disability (20% of hyperactive children are dyslexic compared with 5% of the general population).
- **Dysphasia:** a language disability.
- **Dyspraxia:** when the disorder involves gestures and voluntary movements.
- **Dyscalculia:** an arithmetic disorder; 20% of hyperactive children have dyscalculia compared with 5-8 % of the general population.
- **Dysgraphia:** a spelling disability.

lack of will on their part, but an **inability to concentrate on two tasks at the same time.**

Is academic failure inevitable?

All studies show that ADHD children have a much higher risk of failing than other children of the same age. Around 20% of them have repeated at least one year. This is due in part to their specific learning disabilities, but also a **failure of the school system.** Teachers are not trained for handling hyperactive children; they are not familiar with the disorder and often view hyperactive children as troublemakers who are demonstrating their lack of willpower. Nevertheless, they are also the ones who indicate the first problems children have and are the source of requests for consultation with specialists. If your child is hyperactive, meet with his or her teacher on a regular basis, inform the teacher of the ADHD, ask that a teaching method and attitude be used which are suitable for your child's disorder. It is very important that your child does not feel rejected due to his or her disorder, but on the contrary is understood and helped.

Are hyperactive children less intelligent than other children?

No. All studies show that ADHD children have a normal or even above-average intelligence. They are particularly sharp and curious and their school results are often the opposite of their real abilities. Assessing the intelligence quotient should be systematic when ADHD is suspected, if only to eliminate a mental retardation which in itself could cause psychomotor agitation.

Dyslexia, a more common disorder in hyperactive children

20% of hyperactive children have a reading disability when there are only 5-10% in school population of the same age. Dyslexia is the best known of these reading disorders.

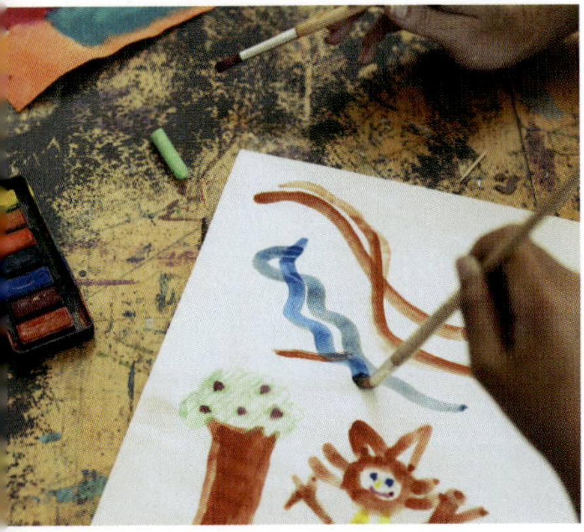

A brain dysfunction

Children are most often discovered to be dyslexic when they start first grade. This particular reading disability has a neurocognitive origin and is tied to dysfunctioning in the brain processes for processing information. Dyslexia causes a real inability to acquire reading techniques which enable the child to learn to read and write, despite having a normal intelligence. This specific reading disability is often associated with hyperactivity.

Recognizing dyslexia

If when reading your child:

- Mixes up phonetically similar letters: m and n, p with b or d, a and an, u and ou, etc.
- Replaces some consonants with others.
- Reverses the order of the letters or syllables or omits certain sounds. For example says "no" for "on" or "arm" for "arms", etc.

And if, on the other hand, he or she does fairly well in arithmetic or other subjects, it is highly likely to find a specific disability to acquire written language, and thus dyslexia. This diagnosis is confirmed by a speech exam. This exam will also eliminate certain pathologies which may cause learning disabilities other than dyslexia *(see box)*.

Dysgraphia, a frequently associated disorder

Dysgraphia is a disorder involving difficulty in learning to write, and is equally frequent in hyperactive children and should be treated specifically by a speech therapist. These children mix up sounds and syllables when writing and speaking. They invert syllables. They have a hard time learning new vocabulary and ignore grammar rules. They do not know how to organize time, and fail to organize a sentence nor do they recognize the different functions of words in the sentence.

How can dyslexic hyperactive children be helped?

Learning disabilities related to dyslexia are accentuated due to attention deficit and hyperactivity. Not only do these children mix up sounds and letters, but they also have a difficult time concentrating when reading, they get lost in the text and lack confidence. They are unable to consistently organize their work (these are referred to as spatial-temporal disabilities). These are some tips to help make learning easier:

- Encourage children when they are successful to boost confidence and self-esteem.
- Separate the work into various short steps in order to best use their attention abilities.
- Set up a work method which gives priority to routine, i.e. have them always work in the same way in order to place emphasis on the content and not the form.

What needs to be eliminated before diagnosing dyslexia

- A hearing disability where language, particularly oral, is distorted with mixing up of sounds.
- A vision disability.
- A simple speech problem.
- An intelligence disability.
- An overall disinterest in learning of an affective origin.

Famous dyslexics

Dyslexia does not prevent learning, nor does it necessarily lead to failure. The following supposed dyslexics should be enough to convince you: Albert Einstein, Hans Christian Andersen, Sir Winston Churchill, Walt Disney, Leonardo da Vinci and Nelson Rockefeller.

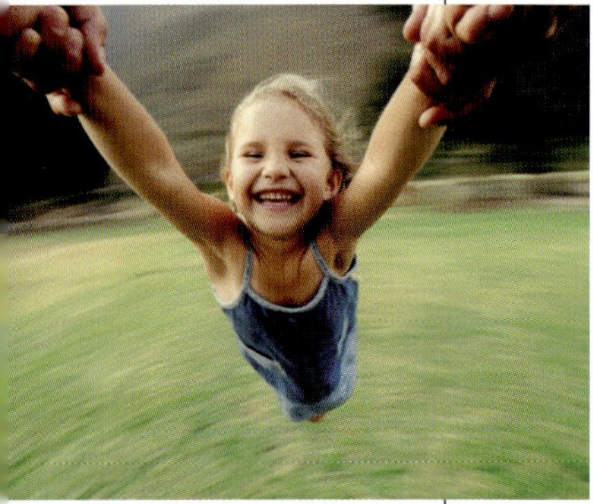

Mood disorders in ADHD

20% of ADHD children will have at least one depression during their childhood, while this figure is only 1% of children in the general population.

Sensitive children

Most ADHD children suffer from their disorder. They are particularly sensitive to their environment, rewards and their failures. Some frequent personality traits in ADHD make them more inclined to mood disorders:

- Being over-emotional and irritable.
- Mood swings, i.e. the tendency to pass from laughing to crying and from anger to calm very quickly.
- Difficulty in controlling emotions, impulsiveness, the tendency to respond immediately to the smallest stimuli without thinking about the consequences of their actions.
- Intolerance to frustrations.

All of these problems make the life of hyperactive children particularly difficult. They are often rejected by other children. The teachers at school do not always understand that these behaviors are due to a disorder. They say that have no willpower, are troublemakers; they are rarely congratulated and punished often. All of this worsens their confidence level and behavior disorders and can lead to a real depression.

Bipolar disorder: a diagnosis to eliminate

Bipolar disorder, previously referred to as manic-depressive psychosis, may start in childhood. It is a mood disorder associated with periods of elation and hyperactivity and periods of depression. In children this disorder causes inattention, impulsivity, hyperactivity, irritability and aggressive symptoms. Thus the symptoms are very similar to ADHD and oppositional defiant disorder; it is sometimes difficult to tell them apart. Often it is a family history of bipolar disorder which makes it possible to make a diagnosis. Making a distinction is of utmost importance since the treatment is not the same for the two disorders.

Signs of depression

Unlike adults, depression symptoms in children are difficult to detect. Actually, children may be depressed without knowing they are because they do not feel sad but "only" misunderstood and alone.

Certain signs should alert all parents to pay attention to their child:

- The child no longer enjoys his or her favorite activities.
- He or she spends a lot of time alone and isolated.
- He or she is more irritable.
- He or she complains of minor disturbances (stomachache, headache, etc.).
- His or her school results are not as good.
- He or she has less energy (this may be difficult to see in a hyperactive child).
- He or she is bored.

If your child has most of these symptoms, he or she may be depressed. To confirm this diagnosis, see a specialized doctor, child psychiatrist or psychologist. You child will be helped by starting psychotherapy or medical treatment in more severe cases.

When hyperactivity is associated with oppositional defiant disorder

Around 20-50% of hyperactive children suffer from associated oppositional defiant disorder. According to DSM IV this disorder is defined as "a pattern of negativistic, hostile and defiant behavior lasting at least six months causing an impairment in social or academic functioning". And this behavior "is not due to another disorder, for example depression."

At least four of the following symptoms need to be present in a child to make the diagnosis:

- Often loses temper.
- Often argues with adults.
- Often actively defies or refuses to comply with adults' requests or rules.
- Often deliberately annoys people.
- Often blames others for his or her mistakes or misbehavior.
- Is often touchy or easily annoyed by others.
- Is often angry or resentful.
- Is often spiteful or vindictive.

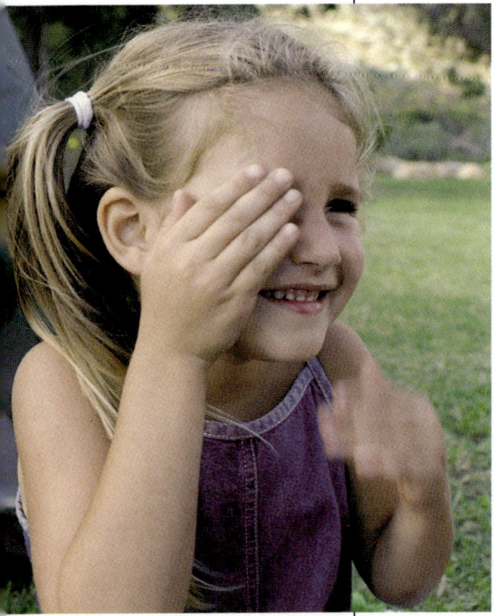

The Tourette syndrome

Described for the first time in 1855 by Dr. Gilles de la Tourette, the Tourette syndrome (GTS) is found in varying degrees in around 50% of hyperactive children while it only affects 5 out of 10,000 children in the general population.

What is GTS?

It is a disorder characterized by tics. More seriously, it is defined by DSM IV as the simultaneous presence of **multiple motor tics** and at least one **verbal tic**. It is a disorder which afflicts mainly males and probably has a neurological origin. The most noticeable sign is the involuntary utterance of obscenities, only present in 10% of cases and thus not necessary for making a diagnosis. Tics are involuntary motor movements which are repeated in a fast and unexpected manner. They occur various times per day, several days a week and must be present for at least six months to make a diagnosis of GTS. The tics may be worsened by stress or anxiety.

André Malraux, a famous GTS

Known for being afflicted with verbal tics and grimaces, André Malraux nevertheless was a great writer and man of action; and he is not the only one. Other famous men had GTS: Mozart, Charles de Gaulle, Émile Zola, Charles Dickens and Franz Kafka.

GTS, a rarely isolated disorder

Most people who suffer from tics also have other symptoms at the same time:

- Attention and hyperactivity disorders before the onset of GTS.
- Learning disabilities such as dyscalculia and dyslexia.
- Obsessive-compulsive disorder (OCD).
- Sleep disorders with frequent waking up and even sleepwalking.

Where does GTS come from?

The exact origin of GTS is not yet known, but hypotheses lean towards a **neurological origin**. Recent research has revealed the role of certain brain neurotransmitters, namely dopamine. Certain studies have discovered that a **genetic predisposition** to GTS exists. In fact, a parent with GTS has a 50% risk of transmitting the syndrome to his or her child. The gene or genes responsible for GTS are not yet known, but research is in progress.

How is GTS treated?

You do not recover from GTS but in debilitating cases it is possible to decrease the intensity of tics using medical treatment. Mainly anti-psychotics are used like haloperidol (Haldol®), pimozide (Orap®) or certain antidepressants (Clorimipramine® and Anafranil®). These treatments work in 80% of cases. In hyperactive children care must be taken because Ritalin®, used to decrease hyperactivity and increase attention, may actually cause tics to increase.

Lots of tics

Different types of tics can be found in GTS:

- **Motor tics**

These can be simple (blinking eyes, tightening abdominal muscles, clearing the throat, making arm movements and head turning) or complex involving various groups of muscles. They are stereotypical involuntary behaviors which are repeatedly reproduced: making different grimaces, touching, squatting, making large genuflections, returning on one's steps, turning around when walking, self-mutilation, etc.

- **Vocal or sound tics**

These are involuntary utterances of words or sounds: clicking the tongue, clucking, grunting, ranting, snorting and coughing. Coprolalia is a complex vocal tic and primarily consists of the utterance of obscene words.

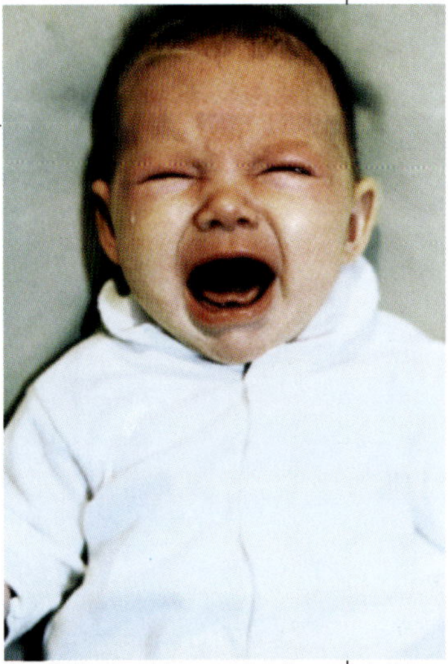

THE EVOLUTION OF ADHD

Hyperactivity in the very young

ADHD often appears before age five. However, in most cases, a diagnosis will be made around age six or seven, when the child starts elementary school.

A difficult diagnosis before age five

Hyperactivity and inattention are very frequent in young children. They are part of normal psychomotor development and are not necessarily pathological. Nevertheless, certain symptoms prior to an actual ADHD diagnosis may be present at that age. However, in young children, the diagnosis is always difficult and the great variation in symptoms requires prudence. Only the evolution and persistence of the symptoms after age seven makes it possible to be 100% certain of the diagnosis.

Hyperactivity is established after two years

Hyperactivity becomes more marked with age which helps in a diagnosis. Certain signs may be a hint: children who have a hard time remaining seated in their chairs, they try to get down or get up by themselves, falling frequently. The same thing happens in a car: they have a problem staying in their car seats, they try to open the door or window, and rarely sleep during a journey.

Why make a diagnosis as early as possible?

Because the brain of a child continues to form during the early years of life and it is easier at that age to change its annoying behaviors. After the age of six it is much harder. In addition, behavior rehabilitation methods are much more effective when started at a young age.

Other behavior signs are frequently associated with this hyperactivity: young hyperactive children frequently lose their temper and are hard to calm down, they cannot stand frustration and have mood swings (fast changes in mood for no real reason). All of these factors in the behavior of children who are also restless may be warning signs of ADHD.

Can infants be hyperactive?

Yes, there are infants who are really hyperactive, even if at that age it is not possible to diagnose ADHD. Often, when the child is older, the parents realize that the infant already had signs of ADHD. The most frequent signs are sleep disorders: these infants have a hard time falling asleep and wake up easily, often screaming. They wake up various times during the night, move often when sleeping, do not nap much and often scream when put in their bed. They suddenly and for no reason change from screaming to being calm. They do not smile much and rarely look at their mothers. When their mothers hold them they squirm and touch everything. They crawl everywhere as soon as it is physically possible. There are also infants who require a lot of attention, who constantly need to be busy and who are stimulated by noise and light. Nevertheless, all these signs are not specific for ADHD, i.e. they may also be present in infants who will be perfectly fine later, or on the other hand be the sign of much worse disorders such as autism.

Ritalin® before age six?

Methylphenidate or Ritalin® is prescribed in children with ADHD after age six. Ritalin® cannot be used before that age. It is actually less effective and has the disadvantage of side effects. There are other central stimulants (for example Dexedrine) which can be given to children starting from age three in exceptional cases. Before age six priority is given to prescribing non-medical treatments: psychotherapy, speech therapy, psychomotility, child-rearing advice, etc.

Hyperactive adolescents

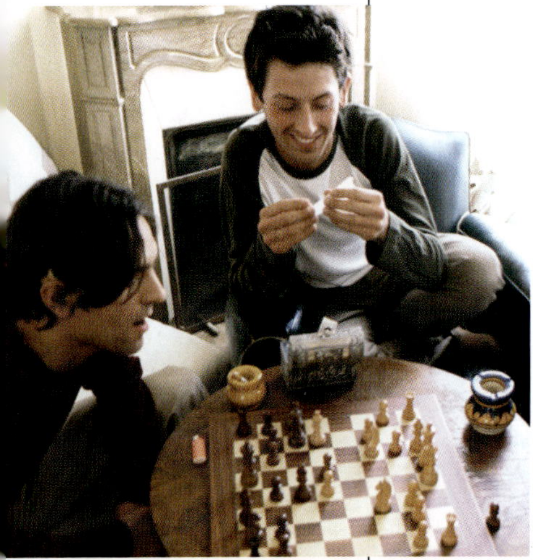

Hyperactivity is not just a problem involving children. Actually, 50-80% children remain hyperactive as adolescents or it evolves into other disorders.

More inattentive than hyperactive

ADHD does not disappear with adolescence, but often changes its form. The attention disorders often become more evident as the hyperactivity decreases. This results in scholastic problems and frequent failures. These **scholastic failures** are worsened by impulsiveness and discipline problems which cause difficulties in relationships with parents or teachers.

Adolescents looking for strong sensations

Hyperactivity is often replaced by an inability to keep still which pushes adolescents to increase their activities and even look for **risky behaviors.** It is also a characteristic of adolescents to look for strong sensations and immediate pleasure. These behaviors are more frequent in hyperactive adolescents than other teenagers. In addition, there are also other disorders associated with ADHD.

Education and ADHD: alarming figures

- 3 times more flunking in hyperactive adolescents compared to adolescents of the same age.
- 8 times more temporary or permanent suspension from school.
- only 65% of ADHD adolescents go to school on a regular basis.
- 25% are in special classes or institutions
- only 22% will go to college compared to 77% of the same age population.

Disorders associated with the main one

Around half of the ADHD adolescents have a behavior disorder compared with 2% of the adolescents in the general population. Impulsiveness, aggressiveness, intolerance to frustration, changes or aggressive action, risky behavior without an awareness of danger and immaturity are the main symptoms. Figures from studies speak clearly:

- 30% drink alcohol regularly.
- 5-30% take drugs.
- 50% smoke cigarettes on a daily basis compared to 24% of non-hyperactive adolescents.
- They have four times more car, motorcycle or scooter accidents.

But this evolution into a **behavior disorder** is more frequent when the hyperactivity was associated with an oppositional defiant disorder in childhood.

A widely variable evolution

Many studies have been conducted in the United States on the evolution of hyperactive children. They have revealed numerous possible evolutions:

- Towards a behavior disorder, the most frequent disorder by far.
- Towards a bipolar disorder or depression, particularly when there has been an episode of depression in childhood.
- Towards an anxiety disorder in 10-40% of the cases studied.
- Towards a social phobia in around a quarter of the cases studied.
- Towards a dependent personality disorder or impulsive personality disorder.
- Towards schizophrenia, very rarely.

Hyperactive adolescents

The manifestations of ADHD in females are not at all the same as in males and this is seen once again in adolescence. Compared to other adolescents the ADHD females start their sexual life earlier and have a higher rate of teenage pregnancy (38% against 4% according to certain American studies). They often use more tobacco or alcohol than other females of the same age which can have detrimental consequences for an unborn child in the event of a pregnancy.

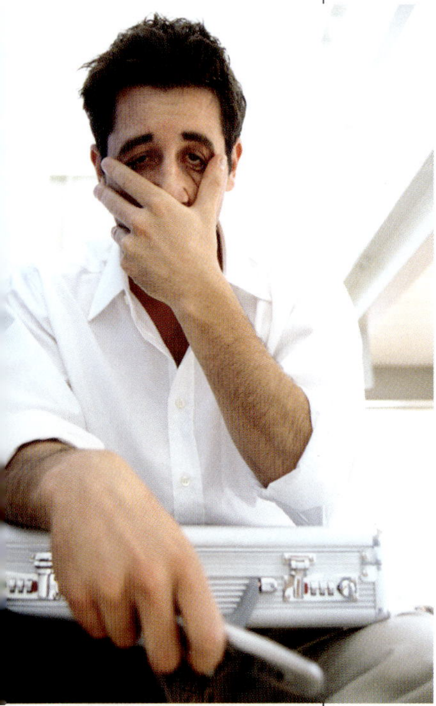

Hyperactivity also affects adults

Out of ten hyperactive children, from three to seven will remain so as adults but with different symptoms. ADHD is not a disorder which starts in adulthood.

An under-estimated disorder

Studies conducted on ADHD in adults are rare and the first article published on the subject is only from 1990. The acknowledgement of adult ADHD in DSM IV only appeared in 1997. This underlines how unknown it is and goes unnoticed in numerous subjects.

Often adults who suffer from hyperactivity seek help for other signs associated with ADHD: anxiety disorders, depression, obsessive-compulsive disorder, chronic fatigue, poor self-esteem, behavior disorders, aggressiveness, alcoholism or drug addiction. These associated disorders are present in 75% of the cases and conceal ADHD symptoms. The diagnosis of hyperactivity is not made and the patients are treated for the associated disorders.

Disorders which can be confused with ADHD in adults:

- Anxiety.
- Depression and bipolar disorder.
- Chronic fatigue.
- Alcoholism and drug addiction.
- Obsessive-compulsive disorder.
- Posttraumatic stress.

(incomplete list)

A difficult diagnosis

Diagnosing ADHD in an adult is never an easy thing. Hyperactivity is never the main problem and the attention disorders often go unnoticed, as the subject does not complain about it. In addition, some pathologies can be taken for ADHD *(see box)* and, vice versa, ADHD can have the appearance of other disorders (anxiety, and bipolar and behavior disorders). According to specialists, two criteria are mandatory to be able to make a diagnosis:

- Finding a previous hyperactivity in childhood, or if a diagnosis was never made, finding behavior suggesting the existence of hyperactivity.
- Persistence in adulthood of attention disorders or hyperactivity associated with at least two of the following five signs: mood swings, intolerance to stress, disorganization, impulsiveness and quick temper.

A suitable treatment

Treating ADHD in adults first involves informing them about the disorder so that they understand that their problems are not linked to a lack of willpower but to a disability. The doctor then establishes a list of suggestions with these patients to help them organize their time in their daily lives: changing pace of life, using an appointment book or lists for daily tasks, getting regular exercise, etc. Associated disorders are treated with specific drugs, which do not have too much of an effect on the patient's life. In terms of Ritalin®, it can be proposed for attention disorders, with the understanding that few studies have been done on its long-term effectiveness and dangers.

Beware of self-diagnosis

When people hear of ADHD in adults for the first time, they often are tempted to discover an ADHD. Who hasn't had concentration problems, anxiety, problems being organized, low self-esteem, a tendency to get bored and chronic fatigue? But a diagnosis is not just based on visible symptoms. A complete medical assessment is necessary. It is not because ADHD is under-diagnosed in adults that it should necessarily be the first thing to think of in the event of psychological disorders.

WHERE DOES HYPERACTIVITY COME FROM?

Is it a genetic disorder?

A genetic component probably exists in the manifestation of ADHD. Several studies have confirmed this, even if the exact mechanisms of this transmission are not known.

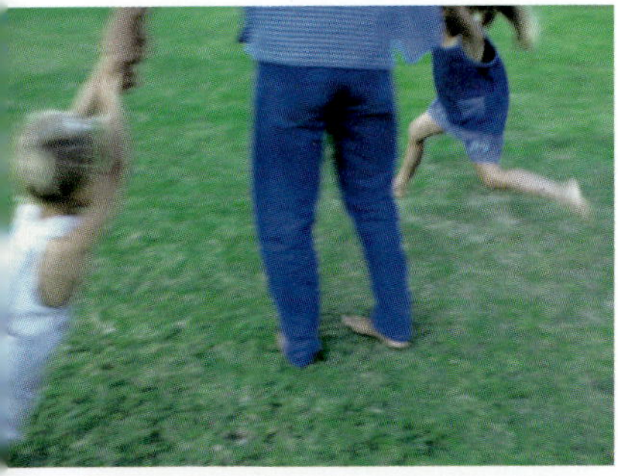

Hyperactive families

All the family studies have shown that ADHD appears with greater frequency in families with a hyperactive person. One of these, published in 1992, examined 140 children with ADHD and 454 of their immediate family members (brothers and sisters and father and mother). The authors noticed that if one of the family members had hyperactivity then:

- The risk of hyperactivity for a female was 6.6 times higher than in the general population.
- The risk of hyperactivity for a male was 1.5 times higher than the rest of the population.

This type of study proves that a **family component** exists in hyperactivity. It can be genetic in origin, but not just that alone. To verify this hypothesis, researchers have used studies on twins.

A particular case: twins

Identical twins have the same genetic code. This means that in the case of a disease transmitted only genetically, if one of the twins is affected the other has a 100% risk of being so. In terms of hyperactivity, studies on twins have shown that:

- In identical twins, if one is affected then the risk for the other ranges from 50-90% according to studies.
- In fraternal twins this risk is around 30%.

These results confirm that there is definitely a genetic part in the transmission of ADHD. Actually, there is a **genetic vulnerability** of being hyperactive and whether this hyperactivity manifests itself or not is based on various factors, especially environmental. Some scientists also believe that there are various subtypes of hyperactivity and that some have a genetic origin and others no. Research continues to discover exactly what it is.

Current research

The most recent studies explore genetic markers. A marker is a particular gene where the presence in the person's genetic code is not due just to chance but is highly associated with a particular disease. Its presence shows the genetic participation in the transmission of the disease.

In hyperactive children two genes have been currently identified as markers: the gene DRD 4 and gene DAT 1. Both of these genes are involved in the production and transport of dopamine in the brain. Dopamine is a molecule which plays a main role in hyperactivity *(see pages 46-47)*.

What is a genetic disease?

Genetic diseases are due to a defect in the functioning of one or more genes. They are hereditary, and transmitted from parents to children. In ADHD, the transmission is autosomal, this means that non-sex determining chromosomes are involved.

The case of adopted children

Studying the presence of a disease in adopted children represents one of the means available to researchers for making a distinction between what is due to genetics and what is caused by the environment where the child is raised. In hyperactivity, this has revealed that a hyperactive person is more likely in the biological family than adopted family of an ADHD child. This confirms the genetic contribution to ADHD transmission.

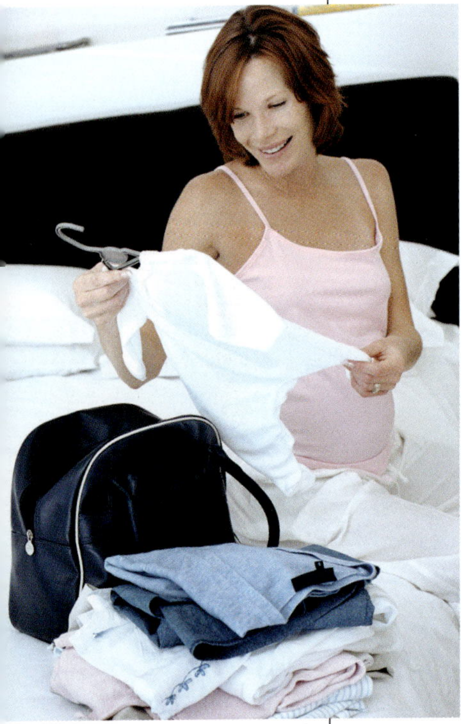

Risk factors

Other than the genetic factors likely to cause hyperactivity, it seems that certain behaviors or events in the life of an infant contribute to increasing the risk of ADHD in children.

Pregnancy, a high-risk period

Cigarette smoking during pregnancy multiplies the risk of having a hyperactive child by 2.1 while drinking alcohol multiplies it by 2.5. These are the results of a study conducted in the United States in 2002 on the smoking and drinking habits of the mothers of 280 hyperactive children and 242 children of the same age without ADHD. Other studies have since confirmed these results. In a more general view, numerous studies have revealed a link between cigarette smoking and alcohol consumption in pregnancy with the onset of mental disorders. On the other hand, no scientific explanation for this relationship has been found to date. So a word of advice: quit smoking if you are pregnant and try not to start again when you have your baby in your arms!

Aside from tobacco and alcohol, other events occurring during pregnancy may cause an increase in the probability of having an ADHD child, however, without being able to pinpoint a direct cause and effect:

- Depression in the mother.
- Diabetes.
- Toxemia.
- Taking toxins or drugs.

- Repeated exposure to toxins: lead, dioxins, pesticides, etc.
- Premature birth or low birth weight.
- Fetal suffering during delivery, pre or post natal complications and perinatal anoxia.

Parents' responsibility

The question of a possible responsibility of the parents in the manifestation of ADHD has been the source of numerous debates among specialists. Some believe that hyperactivity is a symptom that the child has in response to an unsuitable attitude of the parents, for example a postpartum depression in the mother. For other specialists, hyperactivity is a neurological disorder that has nothing to do with affective development. The truth seems less clear-cut. What is certain is that an inadequate parental attitude may worsen a preexisting hyperactivity.

A hyperactive person in the family?

Being the child or nephew of a previously hyperactive man or being in a family where there is already one hyperactive person is the main risk factor. Familial studies have also shown that a family that already has an afflicted member is at a 4-5 times higher risk of having a second member afflicted by ADHD. What's more this is one of the first questions a doctor should ask when meeting restless children with their families.

A higher risk for males?

In all studies, ADHD is more frequent in males. The figures vary from nine boys for every girl, to as low as four to one. According to some doctors, the predominance of males is due to a procedural bias in scientific studies. Males are more frequently diagnosed than females because their hyperactivity is more "disruptive" and causes more trouble at school due to behavior disorders. Females show fewer signs of hyperactivity, but have more significant attention disorders. So females are more afflicted than studies would lead one to believe.

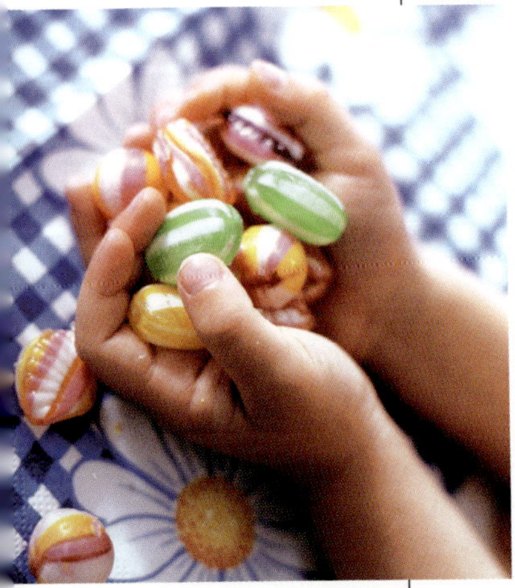

Does diet affect hyperactivity?

Do ADHD children have an iron deficiency?

Yes, according to a French study published in 2004. Researchers analyzed the amount of ferritin (iron reserves in the body) in 53 children with ADHD and 27 normal children. The results are enlightening: 84% of the children with the disorder had a ferritin level lower than normal compared to only 18% of the other children. In addition, the children with more marked ADHD symptoms were also the ones with the lowest levels of ferritin. The link between the disorder and iron deficiency may be related to the production of dopamine. Iron is one of the elements necessary for the synthesis of this intermediate involved in ADHD. It remains to be seen whether an iron supplement would have beneficial effects on hyperactive children.

Numerous studies were conducted in the 1970's on diet and hyperactivity. Many foods such as sugar and certain additives were cited as a cause. But what exactly is the current situation?

Is sugar an enemy of hyperactive children?

Sugar has long been incriminated in hyperactivity. Two hypotheses are the most mentioned:
- Hyperactivity is due to an allergy to refined sugar.
- Or it is due to a hypoglycemic reaction responsible for restlessness and occurring after eating a sugary food.

But these hypotheses were rejected during a study published in 1995 in a major American medical journal. This study reviewed and summarized sixteen clinical studies, and the authors confirmed that sugar does not affect behavior or cognitive performance in normal or hyperactive children.

A diet for hyperactive children

During the 1970's an American researcher, Dr. Ben Feingold, hypothesized that certain foods (chocolate, strawberries, coke and cold cuts) or food additives (flavorings, preservatives and food coloring) could contribute to the occurrence of ADHD in children. This actually involved a chemical sensitization more than a real allergy. But only 5% of ADHD children have this sensitivity to foods. A diet that eliminates all the incriminated foods would decrease hyperactivity but would not have an affect on attention disorders. In practical terms, this diet is hard to carry out and is rarely proposed for treating ADHD.

On the other hand, it is always necessary to make sure that ADHD children have a full and well-balanced diet. Actually, due to their significant motor activity, their dietary needs are higher than those of other children.

Status of iodine in the mothers of hyperactive children

In a small Italian study conducted on 27 females over six years, researchers observed that children whose mothers had suffered from an iodine deficiency in the first quarter of pregnancy are more likely to have ADHD than others. To reduce the risk of ADHD, the group of researchers recommended systematic screening for hypothyroidism (a dysfunction of the thyroid gland due to an iodine deficiency) in women at the beginning of their pregnancy.

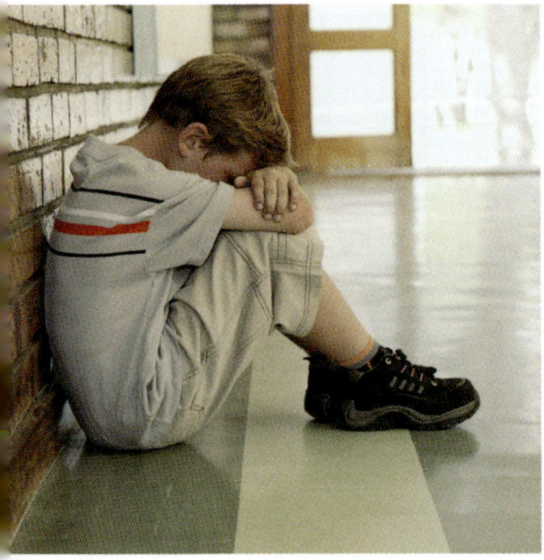

Can ADHD have a psychological origin?

The neurological dimension of ADHD does not exclude the existence of psychological factors and may explain the onset or worsening of this disorder.

Possible psychological factors

Certain psychological factors are found with a higher frequency in the families of ADHD children:

- Depression in the mother.
- Anxiety disorders in one of the two parents, more frequently the mother.
- Marital conflicts.
- Alcoholism in the father.

Nevertheless, it is not known if these factors contribute to the onset of hyperactivity or if the fact of having a hyperactive child causes greater psychological problems in the parents. Nevertheless, if the family environment cannot be held responsible for ADHD in children, it influences how children experience their disorder.

Psychological theories explaining hyperactivity

Psychologists and psychoanalysts have proposed several psychological explanations for hyperactivity.

- The child's instability is an unconscious defense against a separation anxiety from the mother and masks an underlying depression in the child.
- The instability is a psychosomatic disorder, i.e. the direct expression in the body of mental conflicts. These are due to a particular difficulty in managing unconscious aggressive tendencies causing a propensity for action rather than thinking about the action.
- The instability is viewed as a defense against a previous anxiety, i.e. an anxiety from early childhood of which no conscious memory remains.

The family's attitude: a determinant factor

Hyperactive children are hypersensitive and over-emotional children who often have low self-esteem. The role of their families is to support, encourage and praise them whenever possible. A poor relationship with such children may worsen the hyperactivity. If they feel misunderstood, rejected and ignored because of their disorders, the problems will only intensify. Nevertheless, having a good relationship with ADHD children is never easy. If you feel overwhelmed by the situation, it may be useful to see a family counselor. Everyone will benefit from this.

When child-rearing problems are the cause

In certain cases, the family environment is responsible for the onset of behavior disorders in children. This may manifest itself with significant hyperactivity, intolerance to frustration and tantrums, all signs that lead one to think of ADHD. But here the disruption is only a symptom of the child's relationship with his or her parents and often reveals a child-rearing problem (lack of limits and criteria given to the child). To distinguish from real ADHD, the advice of a specialist is indispensable.

Does the mother's attitude have an influence?

A study conducted on mothers in relation to their children of different ages (6 months, 2 years and 6 years) made it possible to uncover some relationship factors between mothers and their hyperactive children:

- A greater frequency of intrusiveness in maternal care (frequent interruptions and physical interferences in the activities undertaken by the infant).
- A certain seductiveness in the mother's behavior (searching for physical contact).
- Over-stimulation of the infant (toys too complicated for his/her age and too frequent verbal exchanges).

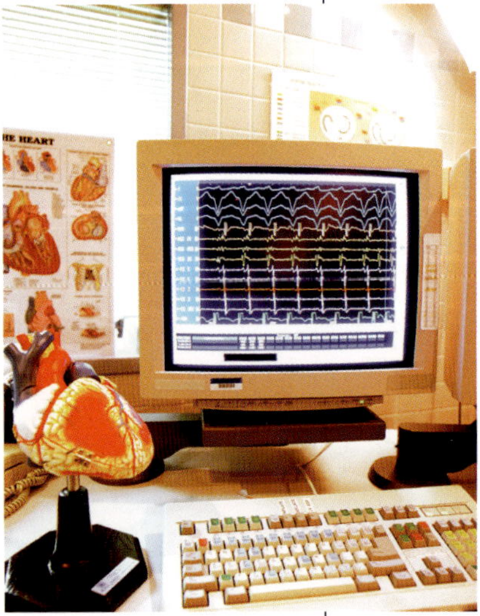

The hyperactive child's brain

Understanding the functioning of the brains of hyperactive children is now possible thanks to the development of new brain imaging techniques.

An organ sensitive to the environment

No two brains are alike just as no two people are alike. Each brain is unique, with its strong and weak points. Aside from the genetic factors which definitely determine most of our behaviors, brain development is also influenced by environmental factors. Moreover, as it develops, minor differences in the environment (mainly the mother's) caused by diet, medicines, hormones, drugs, cigarettes, affective conditions, etc. cause major differences in the brain which has reached maturity. All of these factors modify the way neurons form and connect to each other. The consequences on brain functioning mainly depend on the time when the disturbance occurs. Certain scientists have advanced the hypothesis that these "mistakes" may manifest themselves from childhood, in the form of certain pathologies like ADHD.

A flexible brain?

Cerebral flexibility is the ability of the brain to change due to the influence of past experiences. We are born with a stock of neurons and a number of connections between them much greater than in adults. Actually, all during our lives these inter-neuron connections become specialized: some become stronger, while others disappear based on stimuli from the outside world. For example, children at birth are capable of speaking all languages and pronouncing all sounds but, at the end of ten months of immersion in their mother tongue, they will only be able to pronounce the sounds of the language in which they were raised.

A hyperactive brain

Hyperactivity is due to a failure to prevent unsuitable motor activity. And it is the brain, the organ which controls all our movements and gestures, which is responsible. Current research on cerebral functioning in ADHD children has revealed that specific dysfunctions in certain areas such as the frontal lobes or certain central gray nuclei (for example the putamen) located further to the back. However, in ADHD there is no real injury in these areas, this is why it is referred to as a dysfunction. This is also the reason that no x-ray exists which allows a sure diagnosis. Basically, the child's brain works too well, it overreacts to all sensory, visual and auditory stimuli, without any of the filters which allow non-hyperactive people to function more or less normally.

The brain, an incredible factory

Composed of hundreds of billons of cells which consume 20% of our energy, the brain only weighs 2% of our body mass. It is the backbone of all our behaviors, emotions and activities. The nerve cells (neurons) communicate with each other thanks to electrochemical currents or movements of molecules. Each neuron is then linked on average by ten thousand connections. These are even more numerous and functional when the brain has been suitably stimulated during childhood.

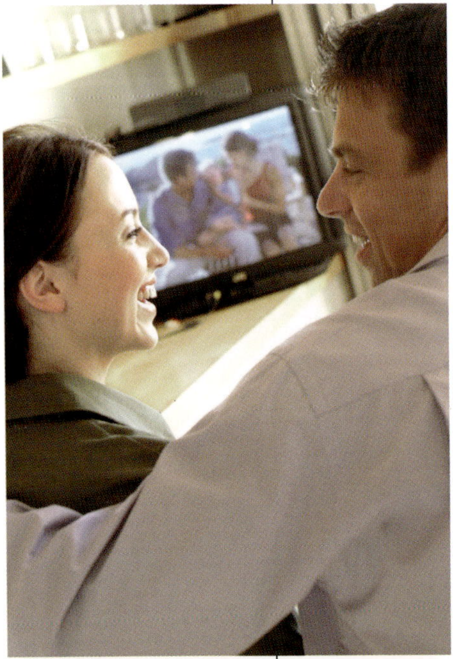

Attention and the brain

It is thanks to the frontal cortex, this area located in the front of our brain just behind our forehead, that we are able to pay attention. This is the particular area that seems to dysfunction in ADHD.

How does the brain work?

Various circuits exist in our brain in charge of circulating information. When we are doing an activity which requires all our attention, these circuits are activated thanks to complex neurobiological mechanisms by making cerebral molecules intervene. These molecules are called neurotransmitters. Thus, we can concentrate on a book we are holding, on our favorite TV show or on a recipe. But these activities require being able **to filter all the foreign information** in our environment. Filtering is the role of the frontal cortex which activates certain neuronal circuits while inhibiting others. Thanks to this information control mechanism, a mother, for example, will not hear thunder rumble but she will wake up at the slightest sigh from her child. It is also thanks to this that we can work

The frontal cortex and its functions

The frontal cortex is a very important area in our brain which manages numerous intellectual activities: organizing the day's schedule, planning how to use our time and defending our ideas with the best arguments. The frontal lobe is equally involved in managing emotions and in what makes up our personality. The rear area, intervenes to control voluntary movements. Lastly, an area located in the left frontal lobe is used to transform thoughts into words.

in a noisy environment without being too disturbed by the surrounding noise. This is called a **resistance to distraction.**

Faulty mechanisms in hyperactive children

In ADHD, there is a **dysfunction of the frontal lobe.** Actually, studies conducted in recent years, thanks to the progress in x-ray techniques, have made it possible to observe a decrease in the activity of this area in children with ADHD. But attention is a complex function in our brain. It also requires the intervention of certain neurotransmitters like dopamine. We now know that these molecules are involved in ADHD. But an attention deficient always has various dimensions. It is not just neurological as pointed out in studies which have not systematically found a cerebral dysfunction; it is also psychological and social. All of these dimensions need to be interlinked for a true attention deficit to occur.

Different types of attention

- **Selective attention**

This is the ability to concentrate on one task to the detriment of another. A deficiency of this type of attention is responsible for a tendency to get distracted and daydream. It is often accompanied by a difficulty in organizing information coming from the environment. This type of attention is the most affected in hyperactivity.

- **Divided attention**

This is the ability to do two tasks at the same time. For example attend a course and take notes or talk and drive.

- **Sustained attention**

This is the ability to maintain attention for a long time. This ability is very weak in ADHD children and also with a lack of sleep.

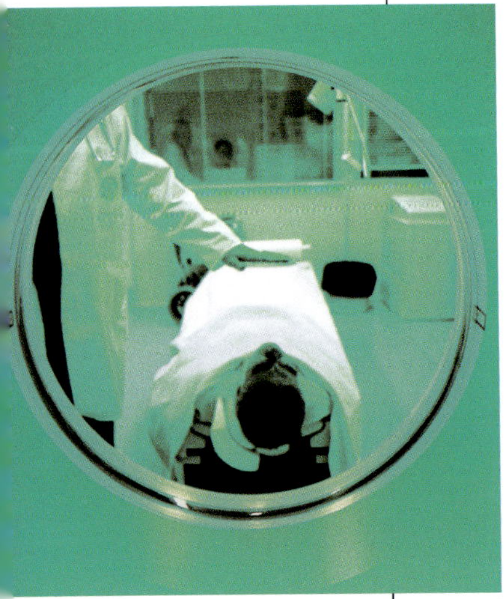

Contribution of neuroradiology tests

Seeing if a brain functions or dysfunctions is now possible thanks to the development of new brain imaging techniques. These techniques have made it possible to better understand the brain's functioning in ADHD.

Analyzing the shape of the brain

Cat scans and magnetic resonance imaging (MRI) are used to see the areas of the brain which become active when stimulated. The centers for language, memory, attention and to control our movements...are thus uncovered. The images are recreated in three dimensions with a computer. These two techniques can be used on children since they do not employ radioactive products. Fewer studies have been conducted on ADHD since the research is recent. Nevertheless, most of them, by analyzing the brain, have shown differences between the brains of ADHD children and those of other children: the right frontal cortex and the corpus callusum are smaller in the former group. However, these abnormalities are not found in all ADHD children and the reason is not yet known.

The effect of Ritalin® can be seen on the brain

The administration of stimulants, like Ritalin®, increases the activity of certain areas of the brain and decreases that of other areas. These are the results of several studies using PET and conducted by researchers on adult subjects with ADHD. However, the effect of this treatment on the brain is not always visible. Additional studies are required to better understand the functioning of this treatment in ADHD.

Analysis of the functions in certain brain areas

Currently used for research purposes, two advanced functional imagery techniques make it possible to view modifications in blood flow in an area of the brain while a certain task is performed, to determine the areas of the brain involved in a certain function. Thus researchers discovered the involvement of the frontal areas in motor and emotional activities.

- **PET** *(Positron Emission Tomography or PET Imaging/Pet Scan)* is based on the emission of gamma radiation emitted by the studied organ, after injection of a radioactive product into them. The radiation is then detected and memorized by a computer to provide three dimension images. This examination can only be performed on adults due to its radioactive nature. It can be used to study the organs, plane by plane, and to reveal the differences in the activation of certain areas of the brain.
- **SPECT** (*Single Photon Emission Computerised Tomography*) measures the blood flow in the brain thanks to the injection of a radioactive product. This technique is used to observe the biochemical and physiological processes as well as the size and volume of the organ. For example, by injecting dopamine marked for a radioactive product, it is possible to view the regions of the brain that use this intermediate.

Discovering the areas of the brain involved in ADHD

As early as 1984, a study of the brain created with SPECT revealed that there was decreased blood flow at the central gray nuclei in people with ADHD. This decrease was due to under activity of the frontal cortex. These results were later confirmed by more recent studies: in 1993, a study with PET revealed a decrease in the consumption of glucose (thus indicating a decrease of activity in the area) in the frontal cortex.

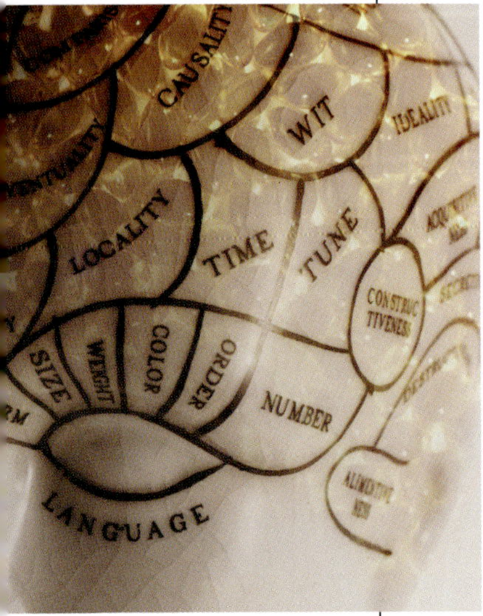

Brain biology and hyperactivity

ADHD may be linked to neurochemical disturbances in the brain. Dopamine is the main incriminated molecule, but it is not the only one.

The brain, a perfected dialogue box

We are permanently in contact with the outside world thanks to our senses (touch, sight, hearing and smell). When one of our senses is activated the information reaches the brain thanks to neurons and is then analyzed there. The information is next transmitted to specific brain centers, based on the nature of the information, before leaving again in the other direction to produce an adequate response.

Neurotransmitters, information messengers

A very important space (and yet very small) exists between two neurons called a synapse. This is where the neurotransmitters are found, chemical substances which ensure communication between two neurons. To go from one neuron to another the neurotransmitter attaches itself to a receptor to cross the synapse with it. For the same neurotransmitter various types of receptors exist which will be activated or not based on the nature of the information to process. These chemical messengers are made by our body from amino acids supplied through food. This is one of the reasons that diet is believed to play a role in disorders related to neurotransmitter production deficits like in ADHD. For example, dopamine is produced from phenylalanine

Differences between females and males: a question of hormones?

Estrogens, the female hormones, may play a role in ADHD which would explain the sex-related differences in the frequency of the disorder. Actually, these hormones interfere with dopamine in the brain, but the complexity of these interactions has not made it possible to understand the exact functioning yet.

(found in chocolate) and tyrosine (present in some types of fish).

Dopamine at the center of ADHD

Dopamine is the most important neurotransmitter of the brain since it represents 80% of the brain's chemical molecules. However, only 1% of the neurons function thanks to it.

Dopamine is involved in many of the body's functions:

- In certain emotions such as the search for pleasure.
- In motor activity and movements.
- In certain basic functions such as awakening, vigilance and hunger.
- In certain behaviors such as searching for reward, sensation and motivation.

Neurons functioning on dopamine are very sensitive to certain situations such as stress and anxiety-inducing situations which will activate it. But they are equally sensitive to experience. Actually, the functioning of these neurons is based on the experiences that the individual has encountered during his or her development. In hyperactive children the production of dopamine is unbalanced which explains most of their symptoms.

Noradrenaline involved in ADHD

Noradrenaline, along with adrenaline and dopamine is part of the family of catecholamines. The effects of catecholamines on the central nervous system are complex and not very clear. Noradrenaline mainly intervenes in mood regulation. In ADHD there is a decrease of the activity of this neurotransmitter in a very special area: the *locus coeruleus.*

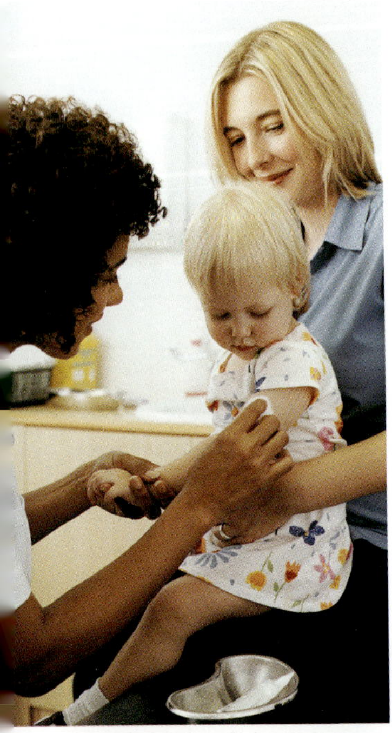

TREATING HYPERACTIVE CHILDREN

Who should you consult?

It is easy to get confused with the great diversity of doctors, psychologists, speech therapists or psychomotility specialists. Who should you consult? Where can you find the most appropriate help for your child? How much will it cost? These are legitimate questions that parents ask when confronted with hyperactivity.

Family physician

Family physicians are a great help because they know the family well, especially the child, and are the first to consult. Their role is to refer parents to a specialist and coordinate the child's treatment. Once a diagnosis has been made, they can ensure follow-up of the children and prescribe Ritalin®. However, a check-up with a specialist is needed once or twice a year.

Child psychiatrists

These are doctors specialized in psychological and neuro-developmental disorders of children. During the first consultation, the child psychiatrist sees the child accompanied by his or her parents to assess overall functioning of the child and his or her family. This is very important to distinguish between a hyperactivity

Specialized hospital services

These are services which provide the evaluation, diagnosis and then follow-up of ADHD children. There are very few and the waiting list is usually long.

They group together all the specialists and thus all the testing is done in the same place, which is very practical and saves time. The evaluation is made in various sessions or, more often, during a day while hospitalized for one to several days.

with a family origin and a real ADHD. These doctors prescribe medical treatments and may also perform psychotherapy of varying types based on their training.

Pediatricians and child neurologists

The pediatrician has a good general knowledge of the children he or she has treated since their birth. Child neurologists are specialized in neurological disorders of children. The consultation revolves around a neurological examination to look for specific signs of ADHD. The pediatrician also looks for the presence of other pathologies such as epilepsy which can be associated with ADHD. He or she is licensed to prescribe Ritalin®.

Psychologists

Psychological treatment is often recommended for ADHD. It is prescribed by child psychiatrists or pediatricians. Psychologists are not doctors and may not prescribe medicines. On the other hand, they make psychometric evaluations (intelligence tests, personality tests, etc.) and perform psychotherapy. Some are specialized in behavior therapies, other in psychoanalytic therapies. A psychotherapy is never contraindicated in the event of treatment with medicines.

Speech therapists

Specialists for oral or written language disorders, they perform a speech examination which is systematically prescribed if there is a suspicion of a reading disability like dyslexia or learning disabilities. Speech therapy is reimbursed in some cases by insurance companies and is prescribed by a doctor.

Psychomotility specialists

These are professionals specialized in the motor development of children based on their psychological development. The psychomotility specialist establishes a test to evaluate the disorders the child has and proposes a suitable treatment. Sessions may be individual or group, generally once a week. In ADHD the work is aimed at fine motor skills, coordination and control of movements.

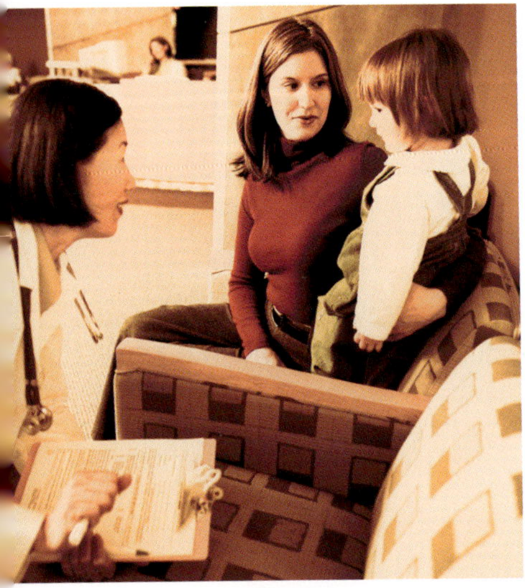

What medical examination is performed when there is a suspicion of ADHD?

Making an ADHD diagnosis requires time and an in-depth medical examination which may require several consultations.

A visit to the doctor

It starts with in-depth questioning even an "investigation" of the child since his or her birth:
- Prior medicines and operations.
- Previous stress or trauma.
- The psychomotor developmental steps of your child.
- An inventory of current symptoms. Everything is taken from sleep to cleanliness, from diet to learning. The questions should provide as broad a view as possible of your child's condition.
- A search for associated disorders such as anxiety, mood disorders, tics, etc.

The doctor will also ask the parents about their own history, looking for previous cases of hyperactivity in the family.

During this first encounter the child may not be restless, often to the great displeasure of his or her parents who are afraid the doctor may not believe them. However, this behavior is frequent in situations where the child is talking to an unknown adult. For this reason the doctor will not be satisfied with just one clinical evaluation. He or she will need to see the child several times, asking teachers for information on the child's behavior at school and sometimes even performing additional tests.

An in-depth medical examination

This includes:
- A complete physical with measurement of blood pressure, heart rate, weight and height (particularly if Ritalin® is prescribed).
- A neurological examination which may reveal minor signs. However, if it is clearly abnormal, another diagnosis should be suspected.
- A vision and hearing test if they have not been done previously.
- An evaluation of learning level based on school records that you bring with you.
- A language, memory, attention and intelligence evaluation using specific tests.

Some ADHD evaluation questionnaires for children or parents, like the Conners questionnaire, help make a diagnosis, but they never replace the clinical evaluation.

Minor neurological signs

Certain minor neurological signs are present in ADHD children:
- Fine motor deficit.
- Stereognosis: difficulty in recognizing an object placed in the hand with eyes closed.
- Prechtl chorea: minor involuntary movements of the hands and fingers which appear in certain situations.
- Synkinesis: existence of associated abnormal movements while making deliberate movements.
- Graphomotor deficit: difficulty with writing.

Setting up treatment

At a later time, the professional will propose a treatment, which can be of different types:
- A medicinal treatment, normally with Ritalin®, if the intensity of the hyperactivity and its negative consequences, namely on learning, justify it.
- A psychotherapeutic treatment for your child, either individually or in a group, with a psychologist, particularly if he or she has psychological disorders associated with the ADHD.
- A speech therapy or psychomotility follow-up.
- Or all of the above at the same time.

The doctor is also there to listen to the parents, inform them on the disorder, and counsel them on the best attitude to have with their child at home and for schoolwork. He or she will answer all the questions parents have, so they should not hesitate to ask them.

Additional tests

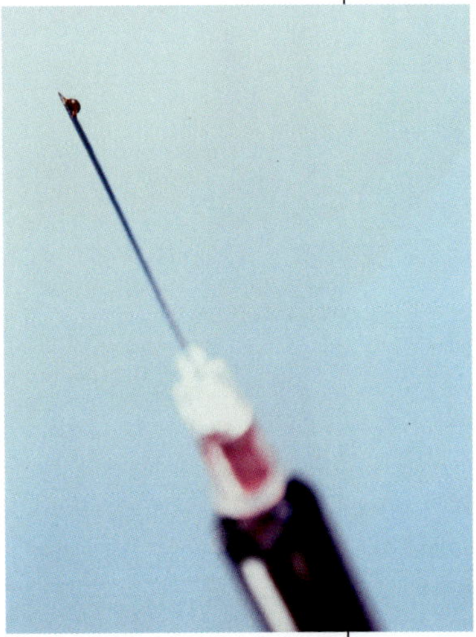

No additional test confirms the diagnosis at 100%. They are performed to have an overall idea of the child's development and abilities, to eliminate other diagnoses which may appear to be ADHD, and to become aware of the situation before starting treatment with medicine.

Three types of additional tests

The tests are not performed to confirm an ADHD diagnosis but to eliminate another pathology which may be responsible for the hyperactivity:

- CAT scan and MRI may be requested to confirm or deny a hypothesis of a brain injury or epilepsy.

- Electroencephalogram if epilepsy is suspected.

- Biological tests: measurement of thyroid hormones to eliminate a hyperthyroidism which may be responsible for hyperactivity and a normal blood test particularly before starting treatment with medicine.

Psychological tests

These are performed by clinical psychologists. Some of them evaluate the profound structure of the personality and may explain the origin of certain pathological behaviors, others examine a particular function such as attention, memory and language. They are used to make a precise diagnosis and to eliminate all other psychological disorders like depression. Psychologists have various tests they can use for hyperactive children:

- Porteus mazes which assess concentration abilities.
- Stroop test which measures selective attention.
- Lowenfeld mosaics used to study personality.
- Rozenzweig picture frustration study which assesses behavior reactions to situations of frustration.

Intelligence tests

The best known is the IQ test. Dr. Alfred Binet is credited with inventing this test to evaluate the intellectual abilities of school-age children. Intelligence tests measure overall intellectual ability, or even partial ability such as practical or verbal intelligence. They can also be used to measure the mental development status in children and thus define their abilities compared to their age level. A result between 90 and 110 is considered to be an average IQ, i.e. the IQ possessed by most of the population. An IQ over 120 is considered above average, below 80 an intelligence deficit. In ADHD, often some minor disturbances are found, even if the intelligence level is normal or above average. Verbal IQ higher than performance IQ, spatial-temporal weakness and graphomotor weakness. However, the idea of IQ tests is very controversial and the results must always be compared with observation of the child.

Is there a test for diagnosing ADHD?

There are dopamine related biochemical abnormalities in the brains of hyperactive children. Researchers have created a radioactive agent, Altropane, which binds with dopamine transporters in the brain. Thus, they are able to use imaging techniques to view the places in the brain where dopamine is missing. This test is currently used for research purposes only and not in practice. It may turn out to be of considerable help in the future for diagnosis if results confirm it.

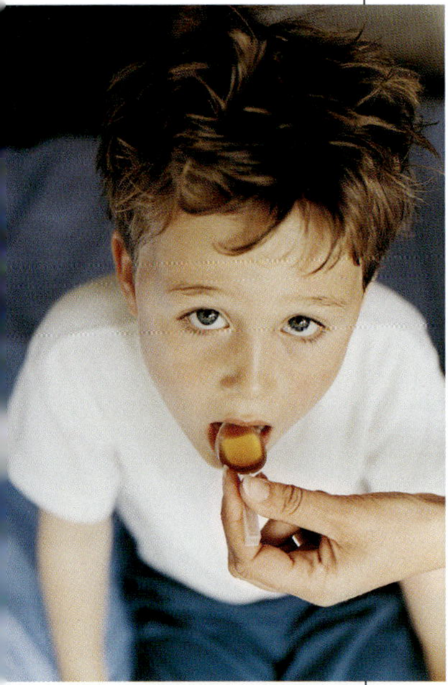

Is Ritalin® a miracle medicine?

Used in most countries of the world for the past twenty years, Ritalin®, or methylphenidate, is THE medicine for ADHD.

The positive effects of Ritalin®

The exact way that Ritalin® acts on the brain is not known, but it seems to have an effect on dopamine and noradrenaline. However, in terms of symptoms, its action is no longer questioned. Parents, teachers and doctors ...all have noticed the effectiveness of Ritalin® on hyperactive children:

- Decrease in hyperactivity and improvement in fine motor skills.
- Improvement in impulsiveness.
- Sharp improvement in attention, ability to concentrate and short term memory.
- Improvement in learning abilities and learning results.
- Improvement in family and social affective relationships and decrease in aggressiveness and oppositional behavior.

However, the results depend on the children. This treatment does not work for some, and the reason is unknown. It seems that the effectiveness is greater in hyperactive children who do not have associated affective disorders (depression or anxiety).

Ritalin® in figures

- 6 million: the estimated number of children taking Ritalin® in the United States.
- 90 %: the percentage of ADHD children treated with Ritalin® in the United States.
- 70 %: the percentage of cases where Ritalin® improves hyperactivity, attention deficit and impulsiveness.
- Several: the number of forms Ritalin® is available in

Not to be prescribed lightly

Despite the demonstrated effectiveness of Ritalin®, prescribing it for children is always controversial. The number of children taking Ritalin® in the United States continues to rise. The pressure from society and particularly schools is stronger and stronger. It is important to note that in the U.S. insurance companies will only pay for this prescribed drug for treating ADHD. Most parents cannot afford psychotherapeutic treatment for their child. Ritalin® is generally prescribed within a overall program for the child, after a rigorous medical examination.

Ritalin® and addiction risk

The opponents of Ritalin® have hypothesized that treatment with the stimulant in childhood increases the risk of adolescent drug addiction. It is important to note that ADHD itself increases the risk of addictive behavior in adolescents and adults. And contrary to these ideas, Ritalin, by decreasing hyperactivity, reduces the risk of this type of evolution.

An overall treatment

The effectiveness of Ritalin® is also greater when it is associated with other therapeutic methods:

- Psychological and educational help for parents.
- Psychotherapy for the child.
- Adaptation of school.
- Psychomotility and/or speech therapy.

Ritalin® has no effect on how the children view themselves. Hyperactive children often have to cope with failures, reprimands and mocking. This can lead to a real depression. At that point help from a psychologist is indispensable.

How do you give Ritalin®?

Ritalin® is never given to children without the parents being worried. However, scrupulously following the prescription directions makes taking Ritalin® danger free.

A dosage adapted case by case

There is no standard dosage. It must be **adapted to the needs and sensitivity of each child.** Normally doctors start with a low dosage (around 0.3 mg/kg) then increased in stages every week until the maximum dose of 1 mg/kg/day is reached. On principle, they always try to find **the lowest effective dose.**

Controlled Drug

Ritalin is classified as a Schedule II central nervous system (CNS) stimulant drug. Distribution is carefully controlled and monitored by the DEA (Drug Enforcment Administration). Because the Controlled Substances Act considers Ritalin a potential drug of abuse, the DEA sets quotas regulating how much can be produced each year. Oral prescriptions are permitted, although a prescription is normally limited to 30 days worth of doses. The use of Ritalin in the US has increased dramatically since 1990. The US consumes 80% of the total world supply and close to 5 times more than the rest of the world combined. Between 1992 and 2000, ritalin production in the US increased 730%. No other nation prescribes stimulants for its children in such volume as the US.

Contraindications

- Absence of ADHD.
- Intolerance to Ritalin®.
- Existence of tics or family history of tics or GTS.
- Certain pathologies such as autism, psychosis or mental deficiency.
- Young women of a child-bearing age.
- When the hyperactivity is due to a lack of child-rearing.

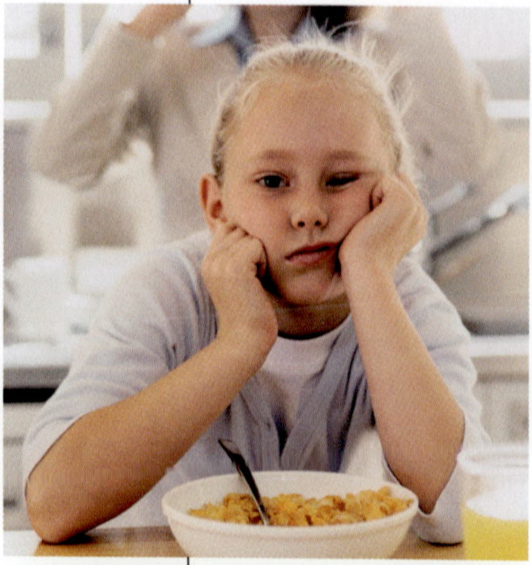

When and how to take Ritalin®?

The effect of a tablet is felt 20 to 30 minutes after taking it and it remains effective for around four hours. Thus it **must be taken at least twice a day** for it to be effective all day. Generally, the treatment is taken in the morning and at lunchtime. It is not given at night to prevent sleeping problems. Another dose can be given around 4 p.m. if the intensity of the disorder requires it.
Ritalin® can be prescribed continuously when the ADHD has serious repercussions on family life, or it can be stopped over weekends, this depends on the child, the severity of the disorder and the family's tolerance.

Who should take Ritalin®?

Ritalin® is prescribed for children with ADHD over age six and with no upper age limit. However, all hyperactive children do not need Ritalin®, far from it. In theory it can be prescribed for adults, but it would be less effective and the side effects would be more frequent.

Significant side effects

- Decreased appetite in 80% of cases but without effect on weight.
- Insomnia.
- Irritability and anxiety, these should cause a doctor to look for a mood disorder.
- Headache.
- Stomach pain.
- Excessive sleepiness is an effect of overdose.
- Worsening or onset of tics particularly in cases of GTS associated with ADHD.
- Tachycardia and high blood pressure in some cases requiring regular blood pressure monitoring.
- Rebound effect when treatment is stopped.
- Slowdown in growth, but with recovery when treatment is stopped.

These side effects are mainly observed in the first two weeks of treatment. They later decrease or disappear.

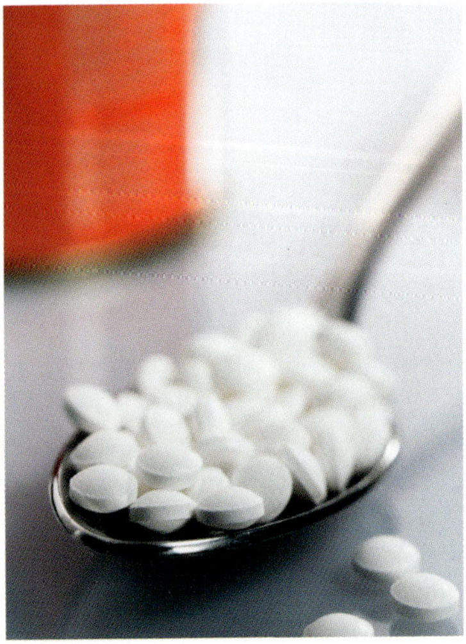

New ADHD medicines

In addition to Ritalin®, four other drugs are mainly used to treat ADHD.

Long acting methyphenidate or Concerta®

This is the **same active molecule found in Ritalin®**. Concerta® is effective for twelve hours and thus can be taken **just once** and acts all day long.
Several studies conducted on six to twelve year old hyperactive children assessed its effectiveness compared to a placebo for periods not exceeding four weeks. Thus the long-term effectiveness of the drug is not known. It is up to the doctor who prescribes the medicine to determine its long-term use.
The most frequent side effects are the same as those for Ritalin®: anorexia, tics, insomnia, headache, irritability and stomach pain. These are found in around 5% of cases, mainly at the beginning of treatment, and generally are not long-lasting.
Concerta® prescriptions must be accompanied by rigorous medical follow-up including clinical evaluation, measurement of blood pressure and heart rate and blood tests (blood count and liver functions).

Atomoxetine or Strattera®

This is the first **non-stimulant medicine** used to treat ADHD. More than two million people in the world have already taken Strattera® and it is available in the United States, Australia, England, Argentina and Germany. It mainly acts on norepinephrine, the chemical molecule supposedly involved in **controlling impulses**, in organization and attention abilities. It can be used for children starting at age 6, and with adolescents and adults are well.
One tablet per day improves the main symptoms of ADHD and **the effect lasts all**

day. It is also effective in children with associated disorders, such as anxiety or tics. Clinical studies carried out on 6,000 patients showed improvements in quality of life, behavior at school and family relationships. The most frequent side effects include: stomachache, loss of appetite, nausea, vomiting, dizziness, fatigue, sleepiness and irritability. The drug company which sells this medicine has also announced that patients who take Strattera® and suffer from jaundice or liver disorders should stop their treatment. This warning was made after two cases of jaundice were observed in an adult and an adolescent treated with the medicine.

Pemoline

Pemoline was sold in the United States under the trade name Cylert®, and in Belgium and in Switzerland under Stimul®. In May 2005, Abbott Laboratories announced that Cylert® would no longer be available in the United States and in October 2005, manufacturers of the generic forms agreed to stop selling them. This action was based on advice from the Food and Drug Administration (FDA) that determined the overall risk of liver toxicity outweighed the benefits of the drug. It was taken off the Canadian market in 1999 due to its liver toxicity. Its effectiveness seems close to that of Ritalin® but fewer statistical studies have been conducted on it. Pemoline is never used as the drug of first choice for treating ADHD, mainly due to its toxic effects on the liver.

Dextroamphetamine

This is a **stimulant** which is part of the amphetamine family. It is sold in the United States and Canada under the trade name Dexedrine®. It does not seem to be as effective as Ritalin® for the treatment of ADHD. It is mainly prescribed when methylphenidate is poorly tolerated or ineffective. This medicine is primarily effective in cases of severe impulsiveness and oppositional behavior. Main side effects include loss of appetite, sleep disorders, digestive problems and addiction. Like all amphetamines this medicine may lead to dependence and a risk of drug addiction.

Less specific medicines

Numerous medicines have been used to treat ADHD with varying degrees of success.

Antidepressants

They are mainly used for disorders associated with ADHD, in particular with depression, anxiety or an obsessive-compulsive disorder (OCD). They are also used when stimulants do not work or their side effects are too negative. However, in the United States some antidepressants are not approved for prescribing to children.

- **Tricyclic antidepressants** (Anafranil®, Laroxyl® and Tofranil®), less effective than Ritalin® based on various studies, sometimes have unpleasant side effects (sleepiness, dry mouth and vision disorders) which may cause the patient to stop treatment. They take a long time to become effective and the effect often decreases after a few weeks of treatment. Their prescription requires medical, primarily cardiac (electrocardiogram), monitoring.
- **Prozac®** (fluoxetine) is approved in the United States for treatment of depression and OCD for children starting at age seven.
- **Effexor®** (venlafaxine) is supposed to be effective for ADHD according to several studies conducted on children and adults.
- **Bupropion**, sold in Canada and the United Stated under the trade name Wellbutrin®, is supposed to be effective for ADHD in adults by acting on dopamine. It primarily affects impulsiveness and anxiety. It can also be found in France under the trade name Zyban®, but it cannot be prescribed for ADHD.

Catapressan® (clonidine)

This is actually a medicine used for high blood pressure. It is effective for ADHD thanks to its **action on adrenaline.** It is generally **prescribed with Ritalin®** to improve its effectiveness. According to studies it decreases the intensity of symptoms by 25-50%, mainly impulsiveness and tics. It has no effect on attention deficit. Thus it is limited to the predominantly hyperactive subtype of ADHD. Blood pressure is the main side effect which requires close monitoring.

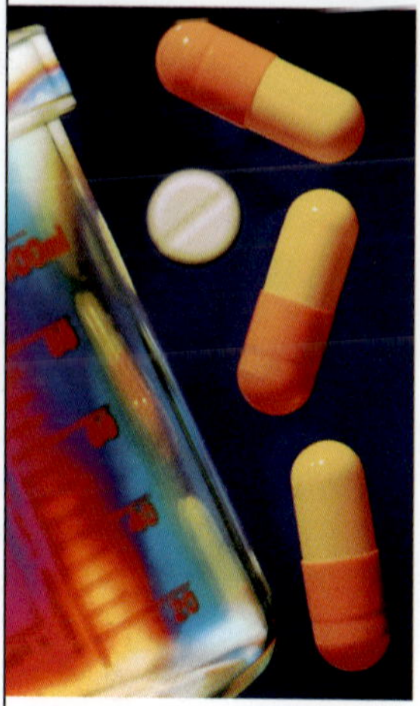

Anti-psychotics (Haldol®, Melleril®, Largactil® and Risperdal®)

These are medicines used for **severe psychotic disorders.** Nevertheless, they are sometimes prescribed for ADHD, mainly if there are behavior disorders (aggressiveness and impulsiveness) and with Tourette syndrome. There are fewer positive effects than with other available treatments and the side effects are worse.

Risperdal® (risperidone), a new anti-psychotic with fewer side effects, is used sometimes with ADHD children for severe behavior disorders, but it is not as effective on attention deficiency. It must never be prescribed as the first treatment.

Mood stabilizers

Normally used to treat **mood disorders**, they have been tried for hyperactive children.

- **Tegretol®** (carbamazepine) is only used for hyperactive children with a history of epilepsy or in cases where other treatments do not work.
- **Lithium** has also been tried but its effectiveness has not been proven.

Natural hyperactivity treatments

Natural remedies are mainly used for moderate cases of ADHD, for children under age six or when parents refuse to use stimulants. But which ones really work?

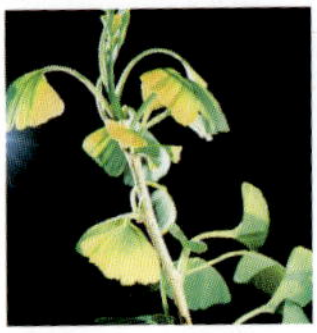

Ginkgo biloba

Ginkgo biloba leaves, from the oldest tree in the world, are known to improve learning abilities and memory by increasing blood flow to the brain. Several studies have shown that ginkgo improves the symptoms of people afflicted with concentration disorders, memory disorders or who are easily distracted. A 2001 Canadian study looked specifically at the use of ginkgo to treat ADHD. For four weeks, thirty-six children with ADHD took a supplement containing 200 mg of *Panax ginseng* extract and 50 mg of *Gingko biloba* extract. An improvement in their anxiety, hyperactivity and impulsiveness was observed in 65% of the cases. These positive effects are due to an increase in blood flow in certain specific areas of the brain. Side effects related to ginkgo are rare (around 0.2% of cases): slight gastrointestinal disorders, headache and skin allergies.

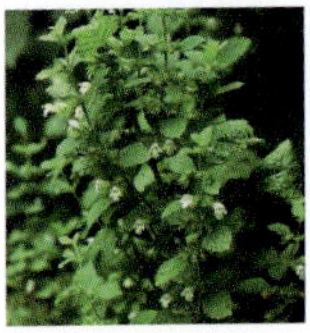

Lemon balm or *Melissa officinalis*

It is used with hyperactive children thanks to its sedative properties. Moreover, it reinforces a substance which is supposedly useful for neuron functioning. However, there is a lack of serious studies demonstrating its effectiveness in ADHD.

Iron

A French study recently revealed that the ferritin level (iron reserves in the body) is lower in certain hyperactive children. Other studies have shown that an iron supplement improves the behavior of hyperactive children and their learning results. An iron deficiency decreases the activity of dopamine in the brain which explains its involvement in ADHD.

Magnesium

ADHD children have lower levels of magnesium than others. A study published in 1994 showed a slight improvement in ADHD symptoms after taking magnesium supplements. However, these supplements are only effective in hyperactive children who have a proven biological deficiency. In this case, the daily recommended dose is around 200 mg/day. Magnesium is often prescribed for states of anxiety and nervousness.

Treatments whose effectiveness has not been proven

- Administration of amino acids.
- Restricting sugar intake.

Zinc

This is a trace element essential for melatonin production, which itself intervenes in dopamine regulation. Zinc acts indirectly on dopamine to improve attention. A 1996 study showed that ADHD children lacked zinc and essential fatty acids. Another study appearing in 1994 was conducted on forty-four hyperactive children between the ages of five and eleven. Half took a zinc supplement (55 mg/day of zinc sulfate). An overall improvement in behavior was observed in this group compared with those who took a placebo. These initial results need to be confirmed with other wider scale studies.

ADHD: treatments which work

• Those which are effective when the hyperactivity is connected to a particular origin:
- Treatment with chelating agent for lead poisoning.
- Zinc, iron, magnesium and vitamin supplements when a proven deficiency exists.

• Those which are effective in a certain number of cases:
- Diet with few allergenic foods for children with a food intolerance (around 5% of hyperactive children).
- Omega-3 polyunsaturated fatty acid supplements.
- Acupuncture: according to a study published in 1998 it is effective in predominantly inattentive ADHD.

Are essential fatty acids useful?

Essential fatty acids are involved in numerous processes in the organism, particularly in terms of good brain functioning. Two omega-3 fatty acids, EPA and DHA, have been incriminated in ADHD by recent studies.

A frequent deficiency in ADHD

Essential fatty acids (EFA) are fats which the body needs to function correctly, but which are not produced by the body: so we must get them from food. The body needs to convert one of these EFAs, omega-3 Alpha-Linolenic Acid (ALA) into two other omega-3 fatty acids: EPA (eicosapentaenoic acid) and DHA (docosahexaenoic acid). Children afflicted with ADHD have a severe deficiency of EPA and DHA. This is the result of a study published in 1995 conducted on fifty-three hyperactive male children compared to forty-three normal children. The fatty acid deficiency in the blood was then associated to the clinical symptoms of this type of deficiency: thirst, frequent need to urinate and dry skin. Other studies later confirmed these results but they still do not know how to explain why ADHD children have these deficiencies.

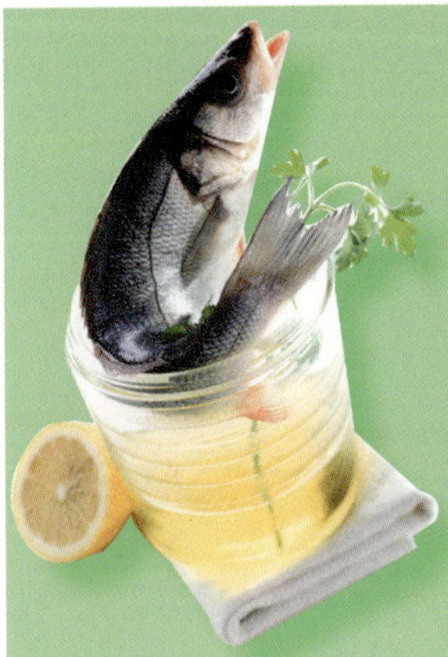

The role of omega-3 fatty acids in the brain

DHA is an essential part of the neuron membrane. Its presence and that of other omega-3 in sufficient quantity is necessary for the neurons to function well. They are involved in communication between neurons and help neurotransmitters (mainly dopamine and serotonin). They are indispensable for the brain development of fetuses during pregnancy, when they are still supplied by the mother. The consumption of omega-3 in the Western population is currently insufficient... this lack may be responsible for neurological disorders like those found in ADHD.

Essential fatty acid supplements: a solution?

The effectiveness of an essential fatty acid supplement in ADHD is still disputed. And actually, the results from different studies are contradictory:

- DHA and EPA supplementation for twelve weeks improves hyperactivity symptoms according to a study published in 2002 conducted on forty-one ADHD children.
- DHA supplementation alone is not effective on ADHD according to a study published in 2001.
- DHA, EPA, GLA and Vitamin E supplementation for 15 weeks improved inattention, hyperactivity and impulsiveness in a study conducted in 2006 on 132 children aged 7-12 years.
- DHA, EPA, GLA and Vitamin E supplementation improved inattentiveness and impulsiveness after 3 months in teenagers aged 12-15 years in a study conducted in 2006.

Thus these results raise more questions than they answer:

- Certain EFA's seem more effective than others for ADHD.
- Certain forms of ADHD seem more sensitive to an EFA supplement.
- The duration of certain studies and dosages used may not be sufficient for revealing an improvement.

Eat some fish!

All specialists agree that our diet should contain more essential fatty acids. According to the World Health Organization (WHO) the daily amount of omega-3 fatty acids is insufficient, and specialists recommend a daily intake of 0.65g - 1 g EPA and DHA daily. Some doctors recommend an amount of 1-2 g per day. Omega-3 fatty acids are found primarily in fatty fish from cold seas. Mackerel has the highest content, followed by herring, anchovy, sardine, plus salmon and halibut. They are also found to a lesser degree in mollusks and

Good omega-3 sources

To obtain approximately 1 g of EPA+DHA and approximately 2 g ALA (recommended daily amounts)

Omega-3 from seafood (EPA + DHA)	**Omega-3 from plants (ALA)**
- 2 oz mackerel	- $^{3}/_{4}$ teaspoon of flaxseed oil
- 2.5 oz of Atlantic salmon	- 3.5 teaspoons of crushed flaxseeds
- 3 oz of pink or red salmon (canned)	- $^{1}/_{4}$ cup walnuts
- 3 oz of sardines	- 2 tbsp of hemp seeds

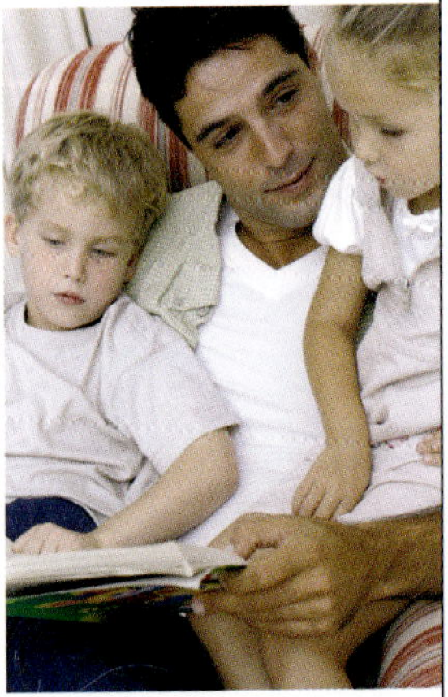

The Padovan method, a new speech therapy tool

Created by Beatrice Padovan, this method associates work on motor activity, verbal activity and thoughts, adapted to the development of hyperactive children. She does this in a very playful way and as pleasantly as possible for the child. During the work, all of the child's key psychomotor development steps are repeated in order to stimulate them. Insurance pays for the sessions in some cases when they are conducted by a speech therapist.

When should a speech therapist be consulted?

One child out of four has a learning disability. In ADHD children this percentage rises to one out of two. These disorders are treated with speech therapy.

Speech therapy is a discipline which works with disorders involving the voice, speech, language and oral and written communication.

Consultation as early as possible

The earlier learning disabilities are treated the better. It should occur if possible in preschool, when the so-called language prerequisites are being taught to the child, meaning the aptitudes needed to learn to read and write. A learning disability can actually be observed at age three, based on information from parents and the teacher.

A speech examination must be systematic in the event of reading disabilities in first grade. In ADHD it is requested when there is a suspicion of dyslexia, dysgraphia or significant learning disabilities. This examination reveals the child's disabilities. It also looks for underlying disorders which may be responsible for learning disabilities: hearing deficiency, neurological disease, psychological disorder and lack of child rearing (child not taught or stimulated). Lastly, it makes it possible to propose a suitable treatment for each child.

Work adapted to the special needs of hyperactive children

Speech therapy must take into account the attention deficit and cognitive disorders specific to ADHD children.

The therapeutic program proposed by the speech therapist will depend on:

- the type of learning disability.
- the age, needs and potential of the child.
- the request of the parents.

In the case of ADHD the speech therapist focuses his or her work on encouraging and making the child confident in order to improve his or her self-esteem.

An effective aid

A speech therapy treatment is used to improve perception, observation and visual memorization skills. It also gives the child strategies to remedy his or her concentration, organization, comprehension and memorization difficulties. This transforms into a progressive improvement in school results, particularly reading and writing.

Psychomotility

Psychomotility is a therapeutic technique which uses the body to access the psyche. It is very useful with hyperactive children when they have motor disorders: clumsiness, coordination disorders and significant motor instability. Psychomotility treatment is generally done at a hospital or treatment facilities since very few psychomotility specialists exist and their treatments are not usually covered by insurance.

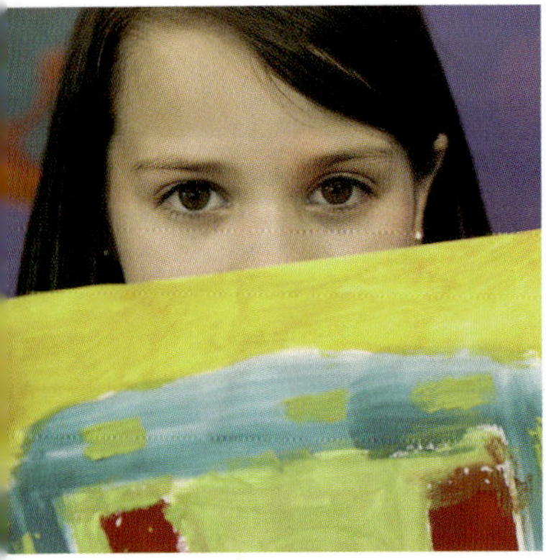

Psychological treatment of ADHD

Psychotherapy includes all the psychological tools used for a therapeutic purpose. Using psychotherapy with ADHD children is always useful, if only to help them to live better with their disorder.

Different types of professionals are licensed to provide psychotherapy. This therapy is generally associated with treatment with medicines in children over age six.

Psychotherapists

This general term describes all those who practice psychotherapy. These professionals may be a doctor or not, or a psychologist or not. There are different types of psychotherapies: family, group, support, based on psychoanalysis, cognitive-behavioral, but also neurolinguistic programming (NLP), transactional analysis, etc. Unless the professional is a doctor, the psychotherapy sessions may not be covered by insurance. For ADHD,

Psychotherapies which work

In a report published in 2004, Inserm (the French national health and medical research institute) analyzed 1,000 scientific studies to evaluate the effectiveness of psychotherapies in children and adults. The main results are shown below.

	CBT	Family Therapy	Psychoanalysis
Depression	+	-	-
OCD	+	-	-
General anxiety	+	-	-
Personality disorder	+	-	+
Autism	+	+	-
Hyperactivity	+	+	-
Behavior disorder	+	+	-

+ = Effectiveness demonstrated

- = Effectiveness not demonstrated or ineffective

only family psychotherapists and cognitive-behavioral therapy (CBT) have proven to be effective *(see the box)*.

Help for the parents as well

A good treatment for hyperactivity should also include help for the parents. This may be done by the family doctor, child psychiatrist or parent associations. It is important that they no longer feel isolated and do not think they are the only ones in this situation. Being informed on their child's disorder will give them the means to cope with it.

Psychologists

These are professionals who have studied psychology at a university level. This education revolves around understanding human behavior and learning different techniques to resolve problems in life. Psychologists practice psychotherapies. They must also pass a specific exam. Sessions with psychologists are not generally covered by insurance and the fees vary widely based on the professional.

Psychiatrists

Doctors specialized in the diagnosis, follow-up and treatment of mental illness, they are licensed to prescribe medicines. They may also practice psychotherapy. The psychiatric profession is disciplined by the specific medical boards. Their services are paid by insurance in some cases.

Psychoanalysts

Generally doctors or psychologists, psychoanalysts subscribe to the theories of Freud or Lacan. They often have specialized training and are under the care of a psychoanalyst themselves. Before choosing a psychoanalyst, you should get information from the various psychoanalyst associations. The analysis sessions are usually not covered by insurance. Statistical studies have not demonstrated a clear effectiveness of psychoanalysis for treating ADHD.

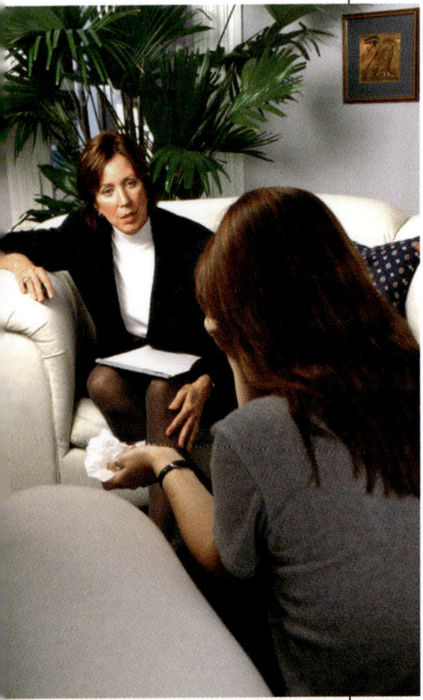

Cognitive-behavioral therapy

The type of therapy believed to be the most effective with ADHD, CBT is based on learning and using new behaviors.

How does the therapy work?

The aim of this therapy is to modify a behavior which is harmful to the person's life. It uses the abilities we all have in order to learn new skills. During the first sessions the patients, along with the therapist, establish what the current problems in their lives are at different levels:

- At a **behavioral level**: hyperactivity for example.
- At a **cognitive level**: "I tell myself I'm worthless".
- At an **emotional level**: "I feel sad" .

Thanks to the intervention of the therapist, the patients' problems are put into context, linked to their personal history. Explanations are made to try and understand the reason the problem appeared or why it continues. After this period of analysis, a particular problem, usually the most overwhelming in daily life is analyzed more in-depth. The patients learn to observe their problem, when it starts, what causes it, etc. Then the patients and therapist discuss the possible goals of the treatment and the means

The cognitive remedy put to the test

This involves cognitive training similar to athletic training: the attention of hyperactive children is stimulated with concentration exercises repeated regularly at home and school. This method lets the subjects acquire new learning activities to make up for the lack caused by ADHD. Different supports can be used such as a computer or audio or visual supports. Recent research conducted in Canada has shown that four sessions per week make it possible to decrease attention deficit and lower Ritalin® dosages.

to put them into practice in order to succeed. The therapist generally proposes specific exercises based on the problem to treat.

How does this help hyperactive children?

The goal is to teach hyperactive children behavior patterns which are better suited to their family, school and social environment. CBT is used to treat the cognitive processes behind the hyperactivity and not the motor agitation in itself. The therapeutic project is tailored to the symptoms which children generally find to be the worst and want to control. The therapist establishes a contract with the children and their families and establishes a program and limits which can be adjusted during the therapy based on the progress made. For ADHD the proposed exercises are mainly aimed at:

- Improving attention and effort.
- Inhibiting exaggerated motor responses based on situations.
- Learning to moderate the level of responses based on requests.

Which disorders does CBT work best for?

- Mood and anxiety disorders: social phobias, single phobias, panic attacks, agoraphobia, stage fright, claustrophobia and depression.
- All other stress related problems.
- Control disorders: tics, tobacco addiction, addiction to gambling, hyperactivity and eating disorders, mainly bulimia.
- Psychosomatic disorders: migraines and chronic pain.
- Certain childhood learning disabilities: learning phobia, enuresis, hyperactivity and social behavior disorders.

Teaching hyperactive children to relax

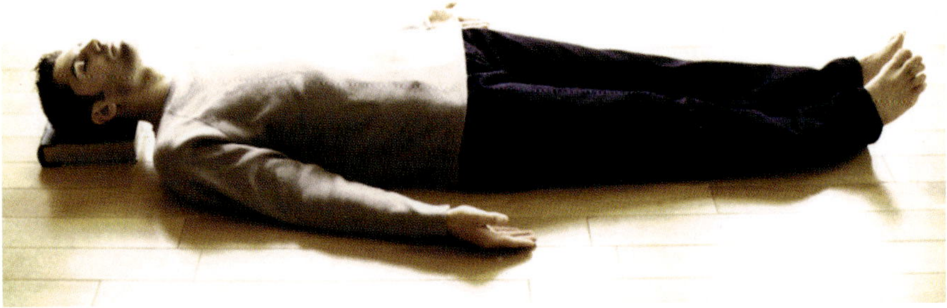

Preparing for a relaxation session

• **Where**? In a peaceful room, warm but not too hot, in the semi-darkness.

• **When**? In the morning to start the day out right; In the evening, after a tiring day or at any time of the day when you feel the need.

• **How**? With comfortable clothes but not too covered up.

- Either sitting in a comfortable chair with arms resting on the armrests, or

- Lying down with your head on a thin pillow.

Hyperactive children are always tense. It may useful to propose relaxation sessions to them which they can repeat at home.

A goal: rest

Relaxation is part of the large family of psychotherapies. The techniques may vary based on the therapist's background but the goal is always the same: learning to relax your body in order to calm your mind. The result is immediate after a session: relaxed muscles, feeling of lightness and peace. Sessions may be individual or group. Relaxation is often proposed for hyperactive children to help them become aware of their bodies in a situation where psychomotor restlessness is not present.

Four steps for well-being

• **You talk about yourself:** all relaxation sessions start with an o**verview of problems.** This helps you to become aware of any current mental blocks.

Talking about yourself prepares you for the session by decreasing tension from stress.

• Learn **to breathe to eliminate stress:** the therapist will ask you to concentrate on your breathing, deep breathing followed by exhaling under the attentive watch of the practitioner. This lasts for a few minutes and prepares your body to really relax your muscles.

• **Think of your body:** once you are completely calm from the breathing exercises, the practitioner asks you to concentrate one by one on the different parts of your body from the feet to the head. The practitioner asks you to tighten and release various muscles one after the other. The therapist helps with this by naming the parts of the body you must concentrate on, using phrases such as "your arms are becoming heavy, heavier and heavier, let yourself go...".

• **Visualize:** this last step is often difficult to achieve when starting relaxation sessions. It involves **making your mind go blank** by getting rid of all foreign thoughts. The therapist asks you to concentrate on a mental image or a color which you associate with something that makes you happy.

The different types of relaxation

In addition to the traditional relaxation techniques, there are some special techniques:

- **Music therapy** uses music to help visualize relaxing images and improves physical and mental relaxation. It is used with hyperactive children who are very sensitive to noises.
- **Relaxation therapy** is a recommended therapeutic method for stress and certain diseases aggravated by stress such as asthma and high blood pressure. It puts the subject into a state of consciousness similar to sleep, to lead the patient to relive painful times from the past and take care of them thanks to deconditioning performed by the therapist.
- **Reiki** is based on the transfer of energy from the therapist to the patient, obtained by the therapist placing his or her hands on the patient's body. The sensations felt are then transmitted to the therapist who analyzes them; this is not used much for ADHD.

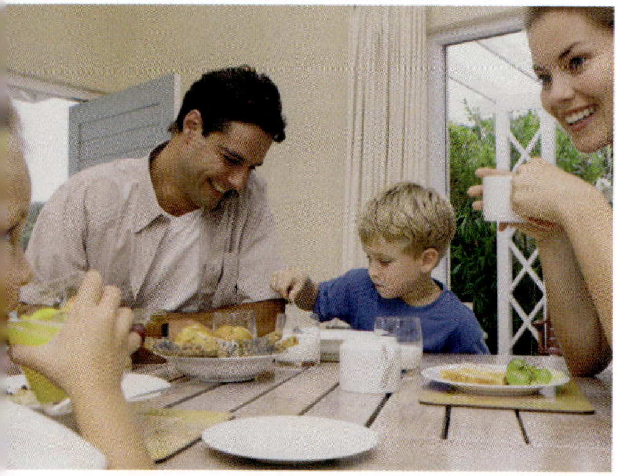

How is hyperactivity managed on a day-to-day basis?

For parents who are tired, infuriated and discouraged by that tornado which is their hyperactive child in the house, here are some tips to help you remedy the above.

Be positive!

First of all change the perception you have of your child:

- Get rid of all the negative adjectives you use to describe your child's behavior and replace them with positive qualities.
- Pay attention to all the things your child does well and not what isn't right and tell him or her about them: hyperactive children are also hypersensitive to encouragement and rewards.
- Accept the fact that it is impossible to radically change your child's behavior. Your child is never going to become a calm and carefree child because his or her hyperactivity is beyond his or her control. Your child is not restless on purpose and is not doing this to "drive you crazy". Even if Ritalin® can help, it never solves all the problems because it cannot be taken twenty-four hours a day.
- Take time to play with your child and show him or her you are interested in what he or she is doing or saying. During these fortunate times avoid giving your child orders, let him or her do whatever, just be there to give a positive attitude to what

he or she is doing. Show your child you enjoy being with him or her. If your child is too difficult or if your child becomes hyperactive, explain that he or she needs to calm down and you do too and that you will start again when he or she has calmed down and then leave the room thanking your child for the time spent with him or her.

Specific child-rearing rules

Hyperactive children are not children like all the others due to their attention deficit, memory disorders and impulsiveness. Many parameters have to be taken into account in raising them in order not to aggravate their symptoms.
Specialists recommend some simple rules:

- Require a minimum of respect from your child for the rules which you have established.
- Set up a list of rules to be followed that you give to the entire family and the adults who take care of your child so that everyone is consistent.
- Collaborate with the school. It is important that the teacher be aware of the diagnosis and if necessary give the teacher information on hyperactivity so that he or she learns how to act with your child; keep track of the situation regularly.

The key to success: a watertight organization

Hyperactive children live in the here and now, this means that they cannot project themselves into the future and have a hard time waiting. They want everything right now. They cannot organize themselves. To remedy these problems they need:
- Life principles and regular schedules for going to bed, eating and napping.
- Simple rules and clear, positive and encouraging reactions.
- Help in organizing their day and activities: if necessary you can write a schedule for the day on a chart that the child can easily check at any time.

Parents: do not hesitate to get help for yourselves

Since hyperactive children are never easy, parents, the mother in particular, may be not be able to take it anymore, become aggressive quickly, be unsatisfied or be on edge. If they are not careful this can turn into a full-fledged depression. Before this happens, you need to be aware that you can get help from a specialist, psychiatrist or psychologist who will listen to you and give you advice, as well as prescribe a psychotherapy if needed.

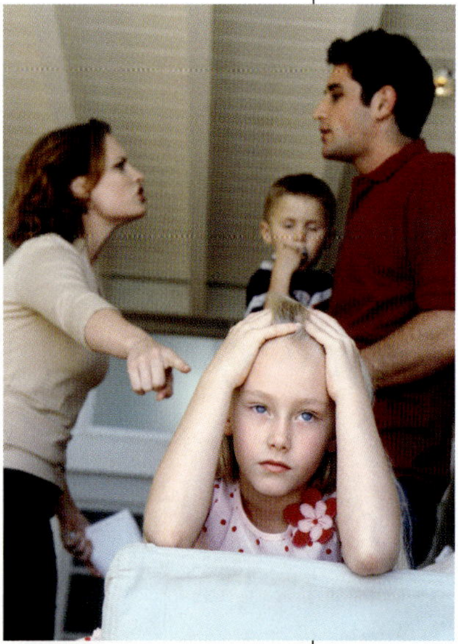

Coping with opposition and impulsiveness

All parents of hyperactive children dream of a miracle recipe for managing conflicts. If one does not exist, there are nevertheless some rules which can be used to progressively improve outburst situations.

Act as a model for your child

You need to remember that children grow by imitating their parents. Before telling your child to calm down, you need to be able to be calm as well. This often means putting some distance between yourself and your child and isolating yourself to calm down and return to your child more serene. This is not always easy to put into practice. To help you, constantly keep these simple principles in mind:

• Conflict in itself is not necessarily a bad thing: don't place more importance on it than it deserves and, more importantly prevent it from getting worse.

• Be positive: children who live in a harmonious environment, where there is not too much upheaval will feel more confident.

Punishing your child: a solution?

Repeated scolding or punishments may lead to a lack of self-confidence in hyperactive children and amplify the problems. However, punishing is necessary to let your child know he or she has gone past the tolerated limits. It must be immediate. Choose punishments which are not humiliating and above all not physical. When punishing your child stay as calm as possible, do not reject your child but briefly explain your reasons. Once the storm has passed do not bring it up again. When it's over, it's over.

How to make children obey

- Tell your child what you want in the form of a sentence and not a question: "Pick up your things, please" is much more effective than "Could you pick up your things?"
- Only ask to have one thing done at a time and make sure your child has done as asked; do not let him or her "off the hook" until it's done.
- Make sure your child has heard what you said, if necessary repeat it or have your child repeat it.
- Give your child time to obey, especially if he or she is busy doing something else: for example you can count to five out loud.
- Set clear limits, which must always be the same and not change based on your willingness or mood.

Managing impulsiveness

Many hyperactive children are impulsive: they do not think about the consequences of their actions before acting. They act carelessly and uncontrollably. So parents have to teach them to control themselves. Some little techniques called mental control may help:

- Ask your child to count to five before doing anything and before answering.
- Ask your child to say the sentence below in his or her head before any risky situation: "stop, think and act".

Pitfalls to avoid

- Feeling responsible and guilty for your child's behavior.
- Being too strict or expecting too much, always adapt to your child's real abilities.
- Not staying in contact with the teacher or, worse, having a poor relationship with the teacher.
- Thinking that you are all alone in this, that your child is the only one who is a problem, when it is common knowledge that hyperactivity is a frequent disorder.
- Systematically arguing with your child, even for unimportant things.

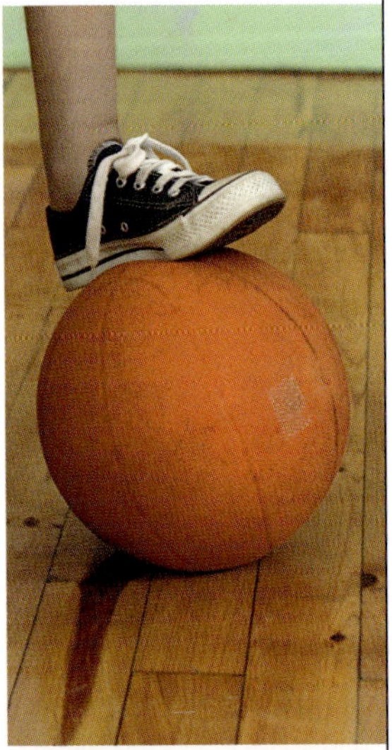

Hyperactive children and sports

Practicing sports is always good for hyperactive children but some activities are better than others.

Practicing sports, a necessity

All children need to practice sports and get exercise. However, for hyperactive children learning a sport implies additional efforts. Efforts involving attention and concentration, in relationships with others and in terms of movements. The most reasonable thing to do is to propose just one activity to them that they really like and keep to it. Sometimes, hyperactive children cannot support the rules necessary for playing a sport. They should not be forced, there is a right time for everything. In this case, you can propose activities without restrictions such as walking, running, picking wildflowers, gardening, sailing, etc.

Don't overdo

Like all other children, hyperactive children get tired when they are stimulated, but unlike others, they do not complain about it. Which means fatigue, irritation, over-emotional behavior, more frequent outbursts and worsening of behavior disorders. It is important not to fall into the trap of wanting to push your child to let off as much steam as possible, under the pretext that he or she is hyperactive or with the aim of achieving more peace at home. This never works. Thus it is up to the parents to manage all extracurricular activities in order to prevent overworking which is always harmful.

Nature and hyperactivity are a good mix

The intensity of hyperactivity symptoms decreases when ADHD children spend time outdoors in contact with trees and grass. These conclusions were reached by a study conducted in the United States on 452 ADHD children from five to eighteen years old. This study also showed that all recreational activities had a positive impact on hyperactivity, no matter what the child's age, sex or social class.

The best activities

Certain sports are more suited to hyperactive children than others. Here is a small list to use as a guideline:

- **Team sports** like soccer or handball which encourage social relationships, involve use of rules and limits and develop concentration abilities.
- **Martial arts** like judo, karate and tae kwon do improve self-control, control of the body and respect for others. It also lets children direct their aggressiveness and manage their emotions while improving motor skills, balance and coordination.
- **Individual sports:** swimming is a source of well-being and calm thanks to contact with the water; horseback riding makes children responsible as they have to take care of the horse and contact with an animal may have a reassuring role in anxious children; skating often appeals to hyperactive children who look for strong sensations, but they must be closely watched.
- **Manual activities** such as pottery, sculpture or making models develop fine motor skills and concentration capacities; they are more likely to be proposed to females which are more inattentive and less hyperactive than males.

Can hyperactive children go to camp?

Certainly! Living in a group situation helps social relationships, learning to respect others and authority, but also implies adding limits and rules for life in a community. Try to find a camp which places priority on creative activities where your child will be able to bloom and gain confidence. Do not forget to inform the people in charge about your child's hyperactivity and explain the rules they need to apply if necessary. Remember to tell them about any medical treatment your child needs to take during the vacation.

Video games, television and ADHD

Many parents confirm that the restlessness and attention deficit disappear or decrease in front of a television screen or video game.

Watching television: not so bad

This is a playful and pleasant way for children to make their memory, attention and cognitive abilities work. Actually, the spectator is not as passive as we are led to believe. Watching a story unfold or a cartoon, starts analysis processes. Children think about what they are watching.

Recent research has shown that hyperactive children watch as much TV as other children of the same age and like the same programs.

On the other hand, contrary to what many parents believe, their abilities to listen and pay attention are inferior to those of other children, particularly when there are distracting elements like toys or other people on the same program.

Too much television increases the risk of hyperactivity

This is the result of a study conducted in the United States that analyzed the television habits of 2,600 children up to age six. Each hour spent watching television between age one and three increases the risk of becoming hyperactive. Three hours in front of the TV per day increases this risk by 30%. These results confirm the influence of environmental factors in the origin of hyperactivity in subjects with a genetic vulnerability.

Video games

Children learn a lot from games. Video games are no exception to this rule. Hyperactive children not only work their concentration abilities but they also learn to control their behavior. Finishing a game session and managing to get to the end, encourages children. They are immediately rewarded for their effort: a good score. However, studies have shown that the performance of hyperactive children with video games is inferior to that of other children of the same age. They are easily distracted, move in their seat and are frequently attracted to whatever is around them. However, these symptoms decrease overall when hyperactive children are enticed by the screen.

The role of parents

Playing as a family lets all the members spend a pleasant time which is much appreciated by hyperactive children. However, it is necessary to limit television with young children: no television under age two, and afterwards no more than one to two hours per day seem to be basic recommendations. Encourage your child to go and get some fresh air if he or she is a video game fan. Your role as a parent is also to guide your children in their selection of programs, taking the contents into account: limit violent movies or difficult subjects for hypersensitive children.

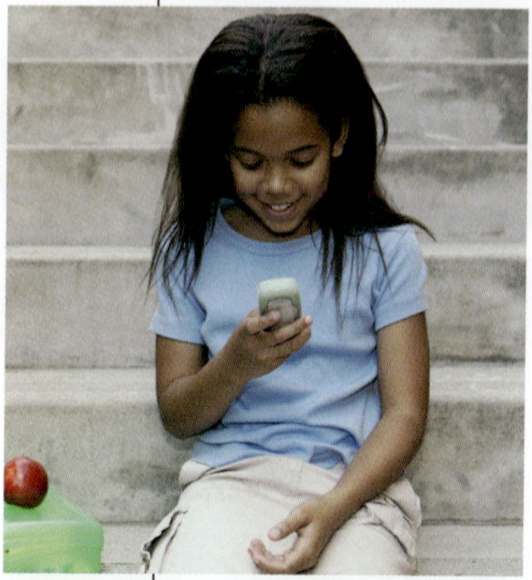

Is music useful for ADHD?

Listening to music may reduce certain hyperactivity symptoms by decreasing stress. Encouraging children to play an instrument is also beneficial to them, all the more so if they love sounds, rhythm and noises. A French doctor, Dr Alfred Tomatis, has also created a therapeutic method using music and sounds. It has had good results with ADHD children. According to the doctor, it is possible to improve attention and concentration using auditory stimulation with music.

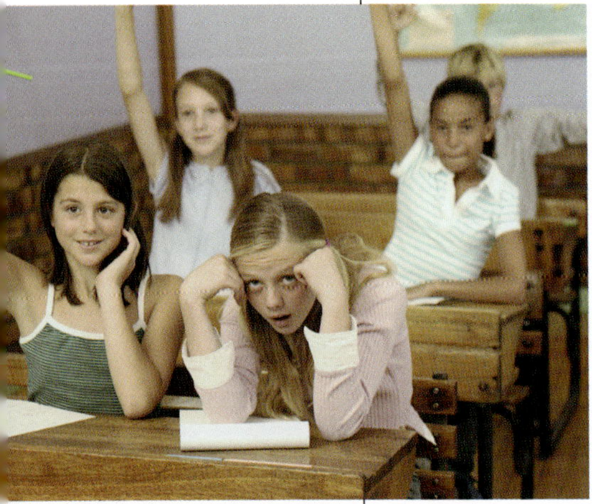

At school

School is the place where hyperactivity is most feared. And yet, it is often at school where the problems of hyperactive children are least considered, due to a lack of awareness of the disorder.

Recess: potential danger

This is a time for relaxing after working hard and the risk for hyperactivity is high. If a child loses control of the situation, you can isolate him or her in a neutral place and explain that it is not a punishment. Talk to him or her calmly and explain the reasons why he or she is being separated from the others.

The place of all dangers

Hyperactive children are often rejected by other children at school and viewed as troublemakers by teachers. There is a high risk that they will feel abnormal, isolate themselves and have a poor image of themselves. This is even more marked if other students make fun of them and if they feel misunderstood by their teachers. All of these factors contribute greatly to failure at school. Thus it is necessary to spot hyperactivity as early as possible, best by preschool age, to quickly start a suitable treatment, inform teachers and decrease the risk of failure.

Adapting the classroom

Avoiding distracting elements in the environment of hyperactive children is essential for encouraging their learning as much as possible, otherwise they will always have their heads up looking at whatever is around them. Here are some practical tips for arranging the classroom:

- The environment must be as neutral as possible. not too many colorful posters on the walls and minimal decoration.
- Keep hyperactive children seated away from windows, in the first row if possible, in front of the teacher's desk and select calm neighbors for them who are not chatterboxes.
- Only let them keep the material they need on their desks, avoid anything extra which is distracting.

Discipline

School is the place where there are the most rules to follow. This is never easy for hyperactive children. They need simple criteria and an adapted attitude. Here are some tips for progressively getting them to follow classroom rules:

- Be firm about the rules to be followed and systematically carry out threats so that you do not lose credibility in terms of authority.
- Avoid getting mad for no reason.
- Never lose sight of the fact that the behavior of hyperactive children is not intentional; this will help you have the most suitable behavior.

How to help hyperactive children with schoolwork?

Since these children are not capable of organizing themselves to do their schoolwork, their parents must help them. Here is an example of scheduling which you can change based on your child and your time:

- Time for relaxing when your child gets home, a snack if necessary, and let him or her let off some steam before starting schoolwork.
- Write the schedule down with various steps if necessary. It is always best to make short steps and divide tasks requiring the most concentration as much as possible, breaks should also be scheduled between the different steps.
- Start with whatever requires the most attention.
- Then stay with your child to make sure he or she is following the schedule and to provide encouragement.
- Refer to the schedule and tell him or her what is scheduled for the rest of the evening.

And do not forget to congratulate your child when he or she has finished because it required much more effort than you can imagine.

How can the teacher help hyperactive children?

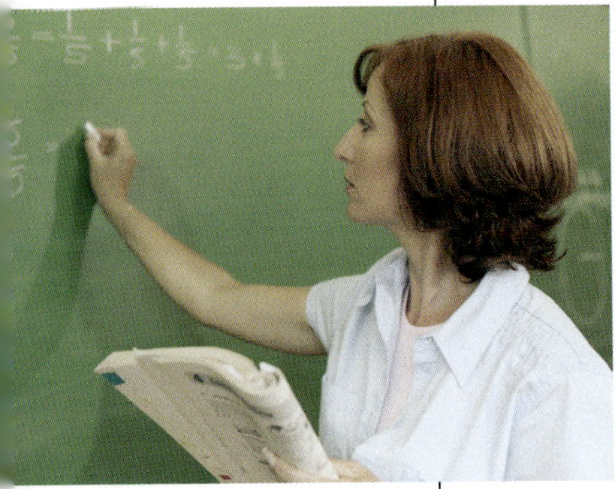

It is imperative that the teacher knows about the hyperactivity. Thus the first thing to do as parents is to inform the teacher of the situation. Then the teacher can adapt his or her methods and the classroom environment to the special needs of the hyperactive child.

Inform, collaborate

Certain practical tips will help teachers with the difficult task of managing hyperactive children at school. Nevertheless, in order to apply them and understand their meaning, the teachers need to understand what attention deficit and hyperactivity disorder involves. Thus, educating teachers is the first priority. However, you must always remember that progress takes time: patience and perseverance are the key words when dealing with ADHD children. Teachers need to meet regularly with parents to assess progress and efforts to pursue.

A customized work method

It is not always easy to treat a student separately and therefore adapting your teaching to the hyperactivity is the key to success. Here are some practical tips to help you handle this type of disorder:

- Only ask hyperactive children for one thing at a time and wait until they finish before giving them more instructions.

- Break down complex or long problems into various steps.
- Encourage students on their strong points.
- Give them a little more time to turn in their work, and ask them to re-write it if necessary.
- Don't try to obtain the impossible. Do not expect well-written work without crossing-out when you know that ADHD children cannot concentrate on the contents and form at the same time.
- Always remember that children with attention deficit must be as active as possible in their learning.
- Propose pair work as often as possible, with the other student checking the work.

Organizing tasks

Helping hyperactive children to plan their day and work is indispensable because they cannot do it themselves. In practice this means having to spend a few minutes with them at the beginning of the day to:
- Make sure they have everything they need close by and only those things.
- Organize their day in key steps which they can later refer to.
- Remind them of certain simple rules to follow.
- Use an appointment book to write down and schedule their significant outings and activities.
- Teach them to always put their things in the same place so they don't forget them.

And at the end of the day you can see what went well and encourage their successes.

Hyperactive children who are liked by their classmates are happier children

In order for hyperactive children to bloom at school and for it to become a pleasure for them to go there, it is important to make sure that they have good relationships with the other children. However, this rarely happens all by itself. Their aggressive reactions and impulsiveness make them unpopular. So it is up to teachers to pay attention to the reactions of their classmates, to teach them how to best communicate with others and to respect differences. Do not hesitate to compliment hyperactive children who make efforts to behave better, in front of the others, to improve their self-image.

Managing attention deficit at school and elsewhere

Concentrating on schoolwork and paying attention to what is said, each everyday task is a considerable effort for hyperactive children.

The importance of self-esteem

Improving self-esteem in these children helps them to cope better with ADHD.

Some tips are listed below to achieve this:

- Never hold back on encouragement, reassurance and congratulations.
- Put qualities and successes before faults or failures.
- Take the time to talk to your child, particularly when he or she is irritated, and propose different ways of calming down (lie down for a minute, breathe deeply, etc.)

Don't ask for the impossible in everyday life

Just because this attention deficit can't be "seen" doesn't mean you should act like it doesn't exist. When faced with children who are in the clouds, daydreamers and distracted it is tempting to say that they do it on purpose, that they have a no willpower and that they need to pay attention. But children with ADHD have an attention deficit that has nothing to do with their willpower. Being aware of the problem, accepting the diagnosis, this already helps these children to feel (finally) understood. Certainly, you cannot recover from ADHD, but it is possible to decrease its impact on daily life and learning by changing your way of doing things.

In the classroom, adapt teaching methods

Parents must absolutely inform the teacher about their child's disorder. The teacher can then use three simple recommendations:

- Encourage the child to correct himself or herself.
- Regularly help the child to keep his or her attention by using a discreet sign you establish ahead of time.

• Children with an attention deficit cannot remain concentrated the entire morning, this is asking the impossible of them. Arrange their schedules so that there are breaks, times when they can let off some steam. Use the beginning of the morning for subjects which require more attention.

• Make lessons lively, give concrete examples whenever possible, illustrate lessons, attention is better when the visual memory is stimulated.

• During the lesson make sure the children are attentive, by calling on them and asking them to repeat if necessary.

• When you want to test them, warn them ahead of time.

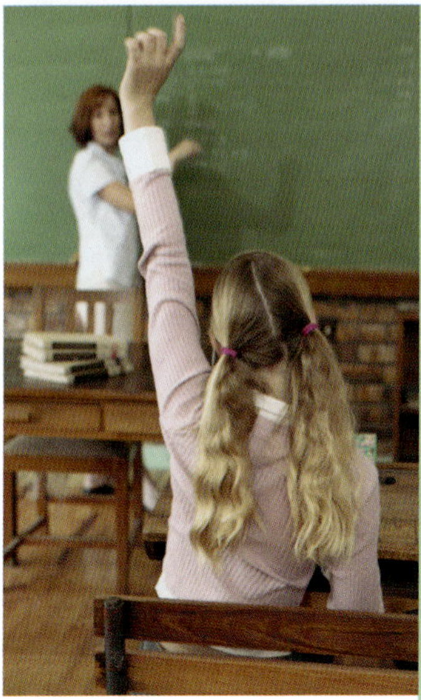

Controlling impulsiveness in the classroom

- Set up simple and clear rules for the classroom. They should be written and put in a practical place where the children and the teacher can refer to them at any time of the day.
- Teach children to wait before answering and to raise their hands.
- Warn the children a few minutes before activities are going to be changed so that they can get ready. Remember that hyperactive children, much more than others, live in the present and are unable to project themselves into the future: it is up to the adult to help them stop one activity to start another.
- If a child's behavior is inappropriate, let him or her know without getting angry, and avoid losing your temper and isolating him or her if the behavior becomes unmanageable. Do not expect perfect behavior from ADHD children, because they just can't do it.

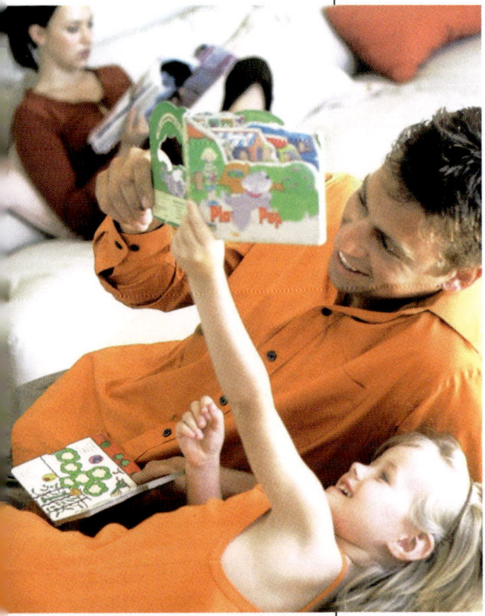

Living better with a hyperactive child

It is never easy to have a hyperactive child in a family. This always requires child-raising adjustments, a way of seeing things differently. The aim of all child rearing is to help the child to understand himself or herself better, to understand his or her emotions to manage them better, to express with words and not behavior what he or she feels and to help him or her live in a social setting.

Hyperactive children have qualities as well!

Put a stop to the list of your child's faults and teach your child to show his or her qualities. A hyperactive child is a child who is:

- Imaginative, inventive, creative, intuitive and not a daydreamer or in the clouds.
- Resourceful.
- Tenacious and not stubborn.
- Sensitive, over-emotional and not irritable and impulsive.
- Lively, expressive and not disruptive.

Looking for lost pleasure

The sensation of pleasure leads to the secretion of certain chemical molecules in the brain called neurotrophines. Recent research has shown that these molecules stimulate neuron growth and increase the number of connections between neurons making learning easier. So stop hesitating: enjoy being together as a family and play with your child without screaming or fighting. Try to create a place so that everyone can bloom, with their faults and qualities. And above all never discourage, even if this requires a lot of effort, perseverance, obstinacy and joie de vivre. This is essential for your child. A happy hyperactive child is a child who feels accepted for what he or she is, understood and encouraged.

Well-considered child raising

Enjoying spending time with your child again means organizing your life around the life of your hyperactive child. So your child rearing principles need to be re-examined. A hyperactive child is not raised like other children. Limits need to be clearly set and written in order to refer to them each time it is necessary. Moreover, they must remain unchanged. This certainly does not mean prohibiting everything, but to select what you feel is the most intolerable. So the challenge is to hold on. A child who does not have limits is a child who does not feel secure. And security is necessary for growing harmoniously.

Parents: be positive!

Thinking positively is not innate, but learned. Here are some things to work on:

- Congratulate your child every time he or she does something well, no matter how small.
- Reward your child when he or she makes efforts.
- Tell your child that you love him or her unconditionally.
- Give your child non-school related responsibilities.
- Create a common project with your child (gardening or cooking).
- Concentrate on your child's strong points.
- Be aware of your qualities as parents but also your limits.

Do not give useless explanations

A child must absolutely feel that the authority of his or her parents cannot be questioned. An order or a "no" must never be argued with. Simply explain to your child the reason for your refusal or order without apologizing. Be patient and tolerant with yourself and your child. Lastly, make sure that the entire family applies the same rules. A child needs consistency in his or her upbringing.

TRUE OR FALSE

Ritalin® must always be prescribed for hyperactive children.

False. Ritalin® is not a miracle cure. Its effectiveness is not 100% and varies from child to child. It is used to treat more severe cases of ADHD, primarily when there are significant problems at school or at home. Psychotherapy, behavior modification, and providing information to parents and teachers are the preferred non-medicinal treatment methods for moderate cases.

It is not necessary to treat the children because ADHD disappears when they become adults.

False. ADHD continues in a third of all cases into adulthood and its frequency is unquestionably under estimated. The typical ADHD symptoms are not as noticeable in adults, and adults often seek treatment for other reasons: anxiety disorders, depression, irritability, sleep disorders, alcoholism, etc. This does not mean that each of these signs conceals ADHD. The presence of symptoms indicating ADHD in a child is a sign in favor of an ADHD diagnosis in an adult.

ADHD is a neurological disorder.

True and false. In around 20% of cases, ADHD does not have a totally neurobiological origin, but is due to other causes: exposure to toxins before birth (exposure to cigarettes or alcohol) or brain damage after birth (infection, head injury or anoxia). It is also necessary to remember that all hyperactivity is not necessarily ADHD. Restless children may be this way for different reasons and an ADHD diagnosis is not usually made until all the other possibilities have been eliminated.

ADHD was discovered a long time ago.

True. The first descriptions of hyperactive children date back to the end of the 19th century, primarily in France, made by Dr Bourneville. However, the first studies on the causes are only from the 1950's. The appearance of the term ADHD to describe certain types of hyperactive children is much more recent.

GLOSSARY

Amino acids: molecules which link together in a chain to form proteins. Phenylalanine is an amino acid.

Agoraphobia: excessive even pathological fear of open spaces and public places.

Catecholamines: a family of neurotransmitters including adrenaline, noradrenaline and dopamine.

Accompanying disorder: association of several disorders or diseases with no causal relation between them. For example, ADHD is often associated with learning disabilities.

Distractibility: trouble keeping attention when there are disturbing elements in the environment. This is one of the characteristics of attention deficit in ADHD.

Dopamine: a hormone in the catecholamine family, produced from tyrosine, an amino acid. It is used to produce other very important neurotransmitters, adrenaline and noradrenaline. Dopamine plays an important role in desire and pleasure phenomena and in movement. Its disappearance in certain areas of the brain is the cause of Parkinson's disease. In ADHD the production of this neurotransmitter is unbalanced.

Dyscalculia: learning disability involving mathematics. It is due to a dysfunction in the logic area and causes difficulty in forming numbers and performing operations with numbers.

Dysgraphia: specific disability in copying written language, without sensory or motor disorder, in subjects with an overall normal intelligence level. It is often associated with dyslexia.

Enuresis: involuntary and unconscious urinary incontinence, like the famous "bed-wetting" of children.

West's syndrome: also called infantile spasms. This generally appears in infants and manifests by brief movements similar to tics, accompanied by muscle spasms for body movements, with high tone.

Fragile X syndrome: hereditary disease caused by a defective X sex chromosome. Afflicted children have a long face, large head, high forehead, thick lips and large ears. It includes mental retardation, attention disorders, learning disabilities and often behavior disorders.

Neuropsychology: a relatively recent science which tends to equate mental processes and the behavior of an individual with the structure and functioning of the brain. It studies mental, cognitive and emotional phenomena in an attempt to relate them to particular areas of the brain. In addition, attention phenomena have been located in the front areas of the brain.

Neurotransmitters: also called intermediates, these are chemical substances produced by neurons (our nerve cells) which ensure communication between two cells. Numerous types exist. The most common are dopamine, adrenaline, noradrenaline, serotonin and acetylcholine.

Toxemia: a syndrome which affects 5% of pregnant women and which is associated with high blood pressure, protein in the urine and swelling. Toxemia can become eclampsia, which is similar to an epileptic convulsion. Fairly rare, eclampsia is equally dangerous for the mother and unborn child.

Serotonin: also called 5-hydroxytryptamine (5-HT), it is a molecule resulting from trytophan, an amino acid. It plays an important role in our mood, sleep, appetite and sexual activity. A serotonin deficiency can lead to depression.

Treatment with chelating agent: treatment for intoxication from heavy metals by using substances able to capture the metal located in the organs and tissues and to bind to them forming a new compound which can be eliminated by the body.

BIBLIOGRAPHY

Studies

AKHONDZADEH S. *Zinc sulfate as an adjunct to methylphenidate for the treatment of attention deficit hyperactivity disorder in children : a double blind and randomized trial*, BMC Psychiatry 2004, 4 (1) : 9.

AMERICAN PSYCHIATRIC ASSOCIATION. *DSM IV, Manuel diagnostique et statistique des troubles mentaux*, 1996, Masson, 4e édition.

BARKLEY R. A. *The adolescent outcome of hyperactive children diagnosed by research criteria: I. An 8-year prospective follow-up study*, J. Am. Acad. Child Adolesc. Psychiatry, 1990, vol. 29, no. 4, p. 546-557.

BARKLEY R. A. *The adolescent outcome of hyperactive children diagnosed by research criteria: III. Mother-child interactions, family conflicts and maternal psychopathology*, J. Child Psychol. Psychiat., vol. 32, no. 2, p. 233-255.

BECK S. J. *Maternal characteristics and perceptions of pervasive and situational hyperactives and normal controls.* J. Am. Acad. Child Adolesc. Psychiatry, vol. 29, no. 4, p. 558-565.

BIEDERMAN J. *Evidence of familial association between Attention deficit disorder and major affective disorders*, Arch. Gen. Psychiatry, vol. 48, p. 633-642.

BIEDERMAN J. *Family-environment risk factors for Attention Deficit Hyperactivity Disorder*, Arch. Gen. Psychiatry, vol. 52, p. 464-470.

BIEDERMAN J. *A prospective 4-year follow-up study of Attention Deficit Hyperactivity and related disorders*, Arch. Gen. Psychiatry, vol. 53, p. 437-446.

BILLARD C. *L'enfant avec hyperactivité. Définition de la pathologie et enjeux thérapeutiques*, A. N. A. E. hors série *L'enfant avec hyperactivité et déficits associés ?* p. 5-6.

CAUSSE-COMBAL C. *Instabilité psychomotrice de l'enfant : analyse bibliographique du concept et étude clinique sur l'évolution à moyen terme des enfants instables*, Thèse de médecine.

MICK E. *Case-control study of attention-deficit hyperactivity disorder and maternal smoking, alcohol use during pregnancy.* Journal of the American Academy of Child & Adolescent Psychiatry, 2002, 41 : 378-85

FINCK S. *Les déficits de l'attention avec hyperactivité : nécessité d'une prise en charge pluridisciplinaire*, A. N. A. E. hors série L'enfant avec hyperactivité et déficits associés ? p. 16-18.

GERARD D. A. *Apport de l'imagerie fonctionnelle dans le THADA*, A.N.A.E., vol. 53-54, p. 116-119.

JENSEN P. S. *Anxiety and depressive disorders in Attention Deficit Disorders with Hyperactivity: new findings*, Am. J. Psychiatry, vol. 150, p. 1203-1209.

KLEIN R. G. *Long-term outcome of hyperactive children: a review*, J. Am. Acad. Child Adolesc. Psychiatry, vol. 30, no. 3, p. 383-387.

KONOFAL E. *Iron deficiency in children with attention-deficit/hyperactivity disorder*, Arch Pediatr Adolesc Med., 158 (12) 605460

LACROIX B. *Approche naturelle du TDAH*, Nutranews, février 2004.

Lou HC. *Focal cerebral hypoperfusion in children with dysphasia and/or attention deficit disorder*, Arch Neurol, 41 : 825-9.

MCARDLE P. *Hyperactivity : Prevalence and relationship with conduct disorder*, J. Child Psychol. Psychiat., vol. 36, no. 2, p. 279-303.

MOREL Y. *Aspects génétiques et moléculaires du syndrome THADA*, A.N.A.E., vol. 53-54, p. 114-115.

PANDIT F. *La prise en charge non médicamenteuse des troubles hyperkinétiques et attentionnels*, Mt pédiatrie, vol. 3, p. 172-175.
Psychothérapies, trois approches évaluées, éditions INSERM, 2004

RAYNAUD J. P. *Hyperactivité de l'enfant : pour une approche pluridisciplinaire concertée*, A. N. A. E. hors série *L'enfant avec hyperactivité et déficits associés ?* p. 27-29.

REVOL O. *THADA : aspects thérapeutiques*, A.N.A.E., vol. 53-54, p. 123-129.

SAÏAG M.-C. ET MOUREN-SIMEONI M.-C. *Hyperactivité de l'enfant*, Encyclopédie Médico-Chirurgicale Pédiatrie (Elsevier, Paris), 4-101-G-92.

VALLEE L. *Hyperactivité motrice et déficits associés : Nécessité d'une approche pluridisciplinaire*, A. N. A. E. hors série *L'enfant avec hyperactivité et déficits associés ?* p. 31-34.

VALLEE L. *L'enfant hyperkinétique avec déficit de l'attention : diagnostic et conduite thérapeutique*, Archives de pédiatrie, vol. 7, no. 10, p. 1111-1116.

WILENS TE. *Bupropion XL in adults with attention-deficit/hyperactivity disorder: a randomized, placebo-controlled study*, Biol Psychiatry. 2005 Apr 1;57(7):793-801.

Books

BARKLEY, R.A.: *Taking Charge of ADHD: Revised Edition*, Guilford Press, 2000.

STEVENS, L.J.: *Twelve Effective Ways to Help Your ADD/ADHD Child*, Avery 2000

SEARS, W. AND THOMPSON, L.: *The A.D.D. Book*. Little, Brown 1998

AMEN, D.: *Healing ADD: the breakthrough program that allows you to see and heal the 6 types of attention deficit disorder*, Putnam 2000

RIEF, S.: *The ADD/ADHD Checklist*, John Wiley & Sons Inc 1997

HALLOWELL, E. AND RATEY J.: *Driven to Distraction*, Simon & Schuster 1995

Additional Information About Attention Deficit Hyperactivity Disorder

CHADD Online (Children and Adults with Attention Deficit/Hyperactivity Disorder)
www.chadd.org
CHADD is the largest national organization for ADHD. It was founded by parents of children with ADHD, and this site has thorough and easy-to-read information for parents about ADHD in children, as well as information about ADHD in adults.
954-587-3700.

American Academy of Child and Adolescent Psychiatry
www.aacap.org/clinical/adhdsum.htm
This site has technical information about the diagnosis and treatment of ADHD.
It describes the current research on ADHD.

National Institute of Mental Health
www.nimh.nih.gov/publicat/helpchild.cfm
This section has a clear summary of ADHD. It gives information on how families can recognize ADHD and get the help they need.

Internet Special Education Resources
Special Education & Learning Disabilities Resources: A Nationwide Directory
www.iser.com/CAADHD.html

Learning Disabilities Association of America
www.ldaamerica.org
412-341-1515

National Attention Deficit Disorder Association
www.add.org
Offers support and information for parents of children with ADHD and adults with this disorder.

Federation of Families for Children's Mental Health
www.ffcmh.org
A National parent-run advocacy and support organization for children and youth with emotional, behavioral or mental disorders and their families.

National Library of Medicine
www.nlm.nih.gov/medline.plus
Free access to Medline, where over four thousand biomedical journals are archived. Click on "Other Resources" and then on "MEDLINE" to conduct a search of articles dating back to the 1960s.

National Association of School Psychologists
www.nasponline.org
Includes numerous tips for parents and teachers on helping children with school related issues like how to manage off-task behaviors, impulsivity, violent behaviors, learning disabilities and how to advocate for your child.